FOWLERS AND WELLS'

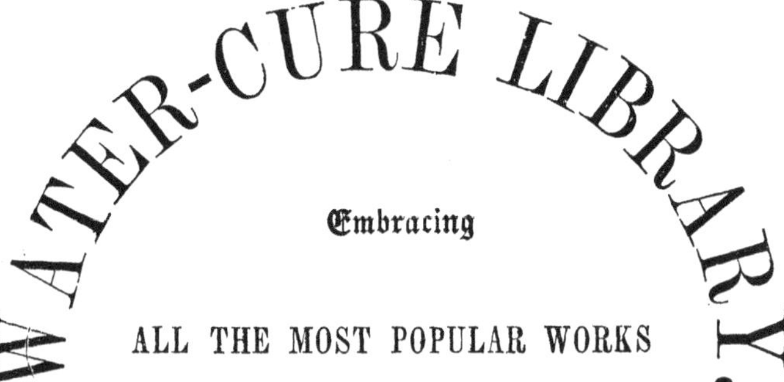

WATER-CURE LIBRARY.

Embracing

ALL THE MOST POPULAR WORKS

ON THE SUBJECT:

INCLUDING:

INTRODUCTION TO THE WATER-CURE;
HYDROPATHY, OR THE WATER-CURE;
EXPERIENCE IN THE WATER-CURE;
THE CHOLERA, AND BOWEL DISEASES;
WATER AND VEGETABLE DIET;
THE PARENTS' GUIDE;
TOBACCO: ITS NATURE AND EFFECTS;
CURIOSITIES OF COMMON WATER;
WATER-CURE MANUAL;
WATER-CURE IN EVERY DISEASE;
WATER-CURE IN PREGNANCY;
HYDROPATHY FOR THE PEOPLE;
ERRORS IN THE WATER-CURE;
WATER-CURE IN CONSUMPTION.

IN SEVEN VOLUMES.

VOL. III.

HYDROPATHY FOR THE PEOPLE;
CURIOSITIES OF COMMON WATER.

NEW YORK:
FOWLERS AND WELLS, PUBLISHERS,
CLINTON HALL, 129 AND 131 NASSAU STREET.
SOLD BY BOOKSELLERS GENERALLY.

HYDROPATHY

FOR THE PEOPLE:

WITH PLAIN OBSERVATIONS ON

DRUGS, DIET, WATER, AIR, AND EXERCISE.

BY

WILLIAM HORSELL, OF LONDON.

WITH

NOTES AND OBSERVATIONS,

BY R. T. TRALL, M. D.

STEREOTYPE EDITION.

NEW YORK:
FOWLERS AND WELLS, PUBLISHERS,
CLINTON HALL, 129 AND 131 NASSAU STREET.
1850.

Entered, according to act of Congress, in the year 1850, by
FOWLERS AND WELLS,
in the Clerk's Office of the District Court for the Southern District of New York.

STEREOTYPED BY BANER AND PALMER,
201 William street.

AMERICAN PREFACE.

On looking over the excellent work of Mr. Horsell, in view of its republication in this country, it occurred to me that a few explanatory and corrective remarks would enhance its value to the American reader. In prosecuting this duty, I found so many topics upon which I could not forbear commenting, that I concluded to supply the editorial matter in an Appendix form, without disturbing the text. One established fact is said to be worth a thousand new theories; yet, for want of ascertained and demonstrable principles, a multitude of truths are lost, or misapplied. If the people can be thoroughly indoctrinated in the general principles of Hydropathy, they will not err much, certainly not fatally, in their home-application of the Water-Cure appliances to the common diseases of the day. If they can go a step further, and make themselves acquainted with the laws of life and health, they will well-nigh emancipate themselves from all need of doctors of any sort. With these convictions, I have commented freely on whatever opinion seemed erroneous, and on whatever fact appeared to be misapprehended. The reader will, I trust, be enabled to bear with me, for speaking so strongly in the mode absolute. Want of room rendered arguments and details inadmissible. I claim, however, not to have taken any position at variance with popular or medical opinions unadvisedly, nor to have asserted any principle without ample investigation.

R. T. TRALL.

NEW YORK, 15 LAIGHT-ST.,

CONTENTS.

CHAPTER I.

CHAPTER II.

CHAPTER III.

CHAPTER IV.

CHAPTER V.

CHAPTER VI.

CHAPTER VII.

CHAPTER XI.

CHAPTER XII.

PREFACE.

One page of personal experience is worth folios of theoretic fancies.—Dr. Kitchener.

Silly, simple, John Bull! why will you pin your faith to fallible or fallacious authority, when you may get the truth so easily by a little personal examination?—Dr. Dickson.

The temperance reformation found me, as it did a large majority of my fellow-men, addicted to the so-called moderate use of strong drinks, which we had been taught to believe were necessary to our comfort and strength, nay, almost essential to life itself. And though I had a good constitution, the excitement occasioned by these drinks, and that arising from preaching eight or ten times a week, sometimes to thousands in the open air, so deranged and shattered my nervous system, and so impaired my general health and strength, that exertion caused me great fatigue. I was constantly troubled with headache and incapacity for mental effort, which I have now reason to believe were increased by the *absurd system of drugging.*

In the year 1833, I signed the pledge to abstain from ardent spirits; and two years' trial proved so satisfactory, that I then resolved to take the second stage in the temperance progress, and to adopt what appeared to me to be the only plan of personal safety,* and also of removing the great curse of

* Alcohol in the human system is an Ishmaelite—his hand is against every man, and every man's hand is against him. Nature tells us plainly she does not need him—that he is her enemy—not one of her principles will sustain the theory that she is benefited by his influence in any form. Every such principle cries out against this abuse—this interference with her operations. Every fibre, and tissue, and organ of the living system sets itself in battle-array against alcohol's invasion, in whatever form he may disguise himself to the eye and the taste.

drunkenness from the land,* viz., TEETOTALISM. I confess I did this with some reluctance, fearing it would injure my health; such were my foolish notions of strong drink. I have since proved that teetotalism "is the first application of science to diet on a large and popular scale," and now sincerely believe that all unnatural beverages might be at once banished from the earth, not only without any loss (except that of disease, crime, and misery), but with the greatest possible benefit to mankind.

For months previously to my adopting the teetotal principle, I had thought I should be necessitated to decline the ministry altogether, in consequence of a settled pain in my left breast; but after three months' abstinence it began sensibly to decline, and in six months it finally left me. My general health improved, and I was enabled to endure much more fatigue, and to do my work with much more pleasure. But still my dyspeptic complaint did not leave me. I was troubled with constipation and headache, especially when I studied more than usual, so that I was under the necessity of taking aperient medicine, never less than once a month, and often once or twice a week.

Soon after the publication of Mr. Claridge's excellent work on Hydropathy, it fell into my hands; I gave it a careful reading, and then a second; I studied its reasonings and facts, and was so fully convinced of the force of most of his observations, that I soon began, by degrees, to adopt so much of his plan as circumstances would admit of, and as I thought my case demanded. Commencing the THIRD STAGE in temperance, I left off tea, coffee, etc., and all hot liquids; also pepper, vinegar, mustard, and all hot spices; took nothing more than

* Lord Althorp told the House of Commons, that drinking intoxicating iquors was the immediate cause of drunkenness. Would you first remove the CAUSE or the EFFECT, if you were aiming at the overthrow of any evil? Philosophy—the philosophy of common sense, says the CAUSE. THEN ABSTAIN. Abandon it, and secure yourself against its bewitching influence.

lukewarm; and generally, *if* I took animal food, I took it quite cold. I rose earlier in the morning; took a cold ablution the moment I was out of bed; rubbed myself dry with a very coarse towel, principally for the sake of the friction; during which, and dressing me, etc., I drank from three to six glasses of cold water. I then took a brisk walk of two or three miles, and returned with a good appetite, to breakfast upon bread and butter and cold water, or Scotch oatmeal and milk. No doubt many of my readers are ready to shiver at even the recital of the above plan; because there are very few, comparatively, who have any idea of the extent of the salubrious effects of water, taken internally, and applied in different ways externally. In the former, this arises from the custom of taking hot tea, coffee, etc., from an early age. The long indulgence of these fictitious habits produces an unhealthy state of feeling, attended with fear that cold water would produce unpleasant sensations, and some injury to the stomach, etc. There is, therefore, a barrier to its use, made up of fear, dislike, prejudice, and custom.* But when this barrier can be leaped over, or broken down, by a little reasoning and reflection, after a few essays, the individual finds that he has been deprived of one of the most powerful conducers to health and longevity, as well as of a great source of pleasure. By the great change produced in the feelings; the greater aptitude for bodily exertion; the marked accession of cheerfulness and gayety, which are the result of a fair trial, all these soon make a DISCIPLE. The increased relish for food, and the quantity that can be taken, and *easily digested;* the light and refreshing sleep, without disturbing dreams; these with the former make a CONVERT. The improved skin and complexion, conferring the freshness of youth; the clear eye, the sweet and wholesome breath: all these united to the foregoing, produce a ZEALOUS ADVOCATE, anxious for others to share his benefits—at least

* A mode of life conformable with nature will admit of no other beverage.

this has been the case with the author of these pages. Besides, arguing the matter merely on the ground of feeling, independent of health and longevity, what can exceed the beauty, freshness, and purity of a glass of cold water, taken fresh from the spring, or from our one-armed friend, the pump? It leaves no mawkish taste behind it; none of those inexpressible feelings which are the results of what is called *good cheer;* but when taken before breakfast, after a bath, or general ablution, it cleanses all the passages, purifies the mouth, and, filling it with sweet and pleasant fluids, makes the individual cheerful, hungry, and wide awake. What a contrast is this to creeping down stairs with the eyes half closed, huddling up to the fire, and swallowing scalding hot tea, etc., eating a few bits of toast, without an appetite, and requiring some relish to make it go down. "We speak that we do know," and that which you may prove to be true, if you will TRY IT.

In consequence of adopting the plan before referred to, I have been enabled to do without the least particle of medicine since April, 1842. Constipation has made its exit, headache and I soon began to be on bad terms, and it threatened to leave me altogether, if I did not, sometimes, treat it with a little tea, coffee, or something more comforting than pure cold water. However, after mature deliberation, I rejected the proffered terms; consequently we parted; and since that time, whenever it makes a call, it finds such a cold reception, that it soon takes its departure.

In all probability it will be thought presumptuous in one unconnected with the medical profession,* to write a book on

* We ask, with Dr. Dickson, "Who will tell me that this kind of study is only proper for medical persons? Who shall say that this description of knowledge may not be made interesting to the world at large?" Without a proper knowledge of the laws of your organization, how can you possibly put in practice the Greek maxim, "Know yourselves." Rowland Hill was no medical man, but as a friend of humanity—a minister of religion—and an advocate for an enlightened view of things, he vaccinated,

health and longevity; but having been extensively benefited by the adoption of the plan he recommends to others, the author thinks he is perfectly justified, nay, called upon, as a philanthropist and Christian, to attempt to lead others into the same paths, knowing them to be safe and happy. While he makes no pretensions to medical science, he hopes he is guided by common sense and a desire to do good. He cannot, therefore, consent to be reasoned or ridiculed out of his feelings and purposes; nor to believe that an illusion, the truth of which has been asserted by some of the most eminent of the faculty, and confirmed by the greatly improved health of himself and of thousands.

In the following pages the author has endeavored to argue the questions at issue, without sophistry, in a plain manner; and he hopes the reader, by trusting to his common sense, and drawing from the facts adduced such conclusions as are obviously inevitable, will be able to distinguish truth from error, and will resolutely choose the former for his guide. We have had enough of fine-spun theories, subtle speculations, and metaphysical disquisitions; we want facts—stubborn facts, for these are the thumb of the right hand in argument. Indeed, there can be no fair arguing without them. They are its basis—its starting point. To this standard we appeal; this is the pedestal upon which TRUTH must stand; because "all those so-called arguments which are destitute of such foundational facts, are not arguments, but only noisy disputes—mere sonorous nothings." To all who can subscribe to this mode of judging of truth, we cheerfully dedicate the following facts and reasonings, patiently waiting their verdict.

As the author's object in the preparation of these sheets was, not *originality* or *fame*, but *usefulness*, he has, in several instances, made use of facts and reasonings which he had met

with his own hands, not less than 100,000 persons, notwithstanding the clamor that was raised against him; being denounced from the pulpit, and insulted by the populace. Doctors have written, and written well, on divinity; and why not ministers write on health and longevity?

with in his course of reading, and which he embodied with remarks of his own, in his commonplace book, without having appended the authors' names; as at that time he merely wrote for his own guidance, and had not the most distant idea of offering his views to the public. Moreover, his desire being to call attention to a subject of vital importance, he thought it was of little moment whether he attained that object by presenting *his* views in the statements of others, or in language and figures which might be more properly denominated his own—believing that the name of an author can give little authority to what may be advanced. Good reasons require no authority, and bad ones derive no weight from any man's authority.

To all who are not familiar with the writings of Hufeland, Claridge, E. Johnson, Graham, Wilson, Courtney, Weiss, etc., it is presumed it will be an advantage to be presented with their views; and even those who are, may be glad to have their memories refreshed by meeting with their old friends, from whose pages we have largely drawn, and who may be read with great advantage. If those who are in the pursuit of health and longevity would purchase the above works with the money they save by giving up all unnatural drinks, etc., and would occupy the time they ought to save from unnecessary and injurious sleep in reading them, they would be *wiser*, BETTER, and HAPPIER. After reading, and carefully studying the above works, those who cannot avail themselves of the valuable advice and assistance of such men as Drs. E. Johnson, Lovell, etc., may, in all simple cases, adopt the plan here laid down for their treatment; and if they will be guided by *reason, nature,* and *facts,* they will have no complicated or chronic diseases to cure.

In conclusion, if these pages should contribute, in any small degree, to afford useful hints, or call attention to this much neglected subject, the author's end will be gained, and his labor amply repaid.

WILLIAM HORSELL.

INTRODUCTION.

Non est vivere sed valere vita.
Life is only life when blessed with HEALTH.

THE present is emphatically a day of *inquiry*. Nothing is now taken for granted. Even children must know *why* certain things are done. Nothing is regarded as being right *because* established, or good *because* antiquated. Every thing must submit to the test of searching investigation; and we see the result of this spirit of the times. Antiquated notions, and established usages and symptoms, are crumbling to atoms. The minds of men are like a great sea, the waters of which are in incessant motion. Science and literature are no longer pent up in a few colleges, royal societies, or inaccessible volumes: from being the greatest of distinctions, they are now become *popular*. Their portals are no longer guarded by a dark phraseology, but having left their retreat, they have begun the work of instructing THE PEOPLE.

It is not only a day of inquiry, but also of *extraordinary activity*. Idleness is neither characteristic of the pious, or the impious—of those who are *really* right, or *positively* wrong. A. Fuller was right when he said, "It is an affecting truth that nothing stands still—all things are at work—in the natural, moral," intellectual, and commercial "world." But if these remarks were applicable to his time, how much more so to ours.* As men

* That these are truly wondrous days, look at that "*great fact*," the *Anti-Corn-Law League*, which aims to increase the size of the poor man's loaf. Last year (1844), they raised £50,000; now they ask for £100,000, and they will get it. The Dissenters' zeal has aroused the Church of England into activity, in the work of education; and her friends have raised near £200,000 for that object, and will yet do much more. The

see and *feel* the force of truth, or what they believe to be truth, they seek with diligence to extend its influence. All are at work, in the church and the world—above and beneath ; and all this various movement tends to universality and diffusion.

Among the other Christian and benevolent institutions of the day, which are the glory of our land, is the Temperance Reformation, which has already, amidst much opposition, accomplished a large amount of good, directly, in the reclamation of thousands of drunkards, and indirectly perhaps still more, in checking the drinking habits of the community. By the multitude these effects have been unappreciated, because to a great extent unnoticed, or if noticed, they have not been attributed to their proper *cause.* But to those who have promoted, and anxiously prayed for, and watched its progress, and been familiar with its multifarious and benevolent bearings, they are palpable and glorious. The general impression against drunkenness has been deepened ; the public mind has been enlightened as to the deceitful and deleterious properties of alcoholic drinks ; genteel society is veering round in favor of sobriety ; and the nation at large is now convinced of the necessity and importance of the Temperance Reformation. Thousands of men, once degraded and wretched in the extreme, are now become sober and happy. Thousands of youth, it is believed, are now so well informed, and so much influenced by

Wesleyans, after raising £221,000 for their Centenary Fund, have now undertaken to provide £200,000 more for schools. The Independents propose to have a day-school attached to every chapel, to accomplish which they have resolved to raise the sum of £250,000 (quarter of a million), in five years. Then comes the Free Church of Scotland, consisting of five hundred ministers, backed by a million of their people, who have spurned the state of yoke, and asserted their claim to perfect liberty of conscience. They have already raised £200,000 to build places of worship ; £100,000 more for the support of their ministers ; and now they ask the religious world to assist them to raise £300,000 more. What do these facts betoken, but *earnestness, power,* and *intelligence* in the people, such as was never before known ? And the ends are even more noble than the means ; they are *Freedom, Knowledge,* and *Religion.*

temperance proceedings, that they are not very likely to fall in the snare of their fathers. Thousands of families, once desolated and despised, and upon the verge of ruin, are now well provided for, united, and happy. Many neighborhoods, once noted for disorder, riot, and immorality, are now peaceable and quiet. Many places of worship, once comparatively empty, are now frequented by numbers of reformed characters, hearing the word of life. And of these there are hundreds, who were once like the man among the tombs, cutting themselves, who are now clothed, and in their right mind, sitting at the feet of Jesus. It has also given rise to several valuable institutions, such as the *Independent Order of Rechabites,** a first-rate benefit society, consisting of a noble army of "life-guards" of our temperance rights, thirty thousand strong, and still increasing (see Appendix, A.); the *United Order of Female Rechabites,* consisting of five hundred tents; besides a goodly number of juvenile male and female tents, composed of children, who are the hope of the world. Then comes the *Temperance Providence Institution,*† which has already issued more than one thousand policies—a proof of the estimation in which it is held by the temperance public, for whose benefit it was established; also the *Temperance Emigrant Society,*‡ estab-

* See Rules, which can be had of any of the members, some of whom are to be found in most towns. Their Monthly Magazine is one of the best and cheapest of our temperance publications, and can be had of any bookseller—of Houlston, Paternoster Row.

† Their office is 39 Moorgate-st., London. The Third Annual Report of this society may now be had (gratis) on application, with tracts explaining the benefit of Life Assurance. The brilliant success of this institution, and the remarkable exemption from loss which it has enjoyed, justify us in urging upon the friends of temperance the *duty,* as well as *desirableness,* of securing a share in its benefits. We *urge* upon every teetotaler the importance of getting full information immediately, which will be most obligingly given by the secretary, Theo. Compton, Esq., F.S.S.

‡ A *share* in the above society entitles the holder thereof to eighty acres of land, a house to live in (having more conveniences in it than one for which a person must give £10 per annum in London or Liverpool), and

lished in Liverpool, under the patronage of L. Heyworth, Esq.—a guaranty for its respectability, as is also the moral and religious character of its secretary, Mr. R. Gorst. They have now numbers subscribing for 30,080 acres of land, which will be their own property, and their heirs, forever. The *Temperance Building Societies,** designed to assist every teetotaler to become his own landlord, and thus furnish *homes for the people.* And lastly, though not least, it has given rise to a spirit of inquiry into the various branches of *physical science,* and led thousands, who previously disregarded the laws of health, to read, think, examine, and practice them. This is a natural consequence of an enlightened adoption of our views; and in proportion as this spirit is cultivated, will be the permanency and success of our operations. We do not say that the preservation of health, and the attainment of longevity, are the only motives by which temperance men will be influenced; there are various and important benefits of a pecuniary, moral, and religious character, which also operate upon their minds, and regulate their conduct. But we do insist upon the im-

£9 5*s.* in cash, or with its worth in goods. The entrance is two shillings and sixpence, and the subscription one shilling per week, per share. Prospectuses may be had, gratis; likewise the laws of the society, price sixpence; and a pamphlet giving a description of *Wisconsin,* in the *United States.* Their agent is gone out to this place, to purchase and prepare the land, build the houses, and make the necessary arrangements for the reception of the first portion of emigrants, which left England in April (1844). For further information, prospectus, rules, etc., apply to the secretary, Temperance Hotel, 17 Bulton-st., Liverpool.

* The first, second, and third are established at Hart's Temperance Hotel, 159 Aldersgate-st., London; the South London, at the Temperance Hall, Waterloo Road—E. R. Mesban, secretary, 6 Fleming-st., Kingsland Road, London. The entrance money varies, but the monthly subscription is ten shillings per share. Members may increase the number of their shares at any time, without any extra entrance money. The association is to continue in existence until every unadvanced share becomes of the value of £120, which it is fully expected will be in ten years, or less. For prospectuses, etc., gratis, apply (if by letter post-paid, with stamp for reply) to the secretary, J. R. Macarthur 3 Taymouth Terrace, London Hospital, London.

portance of considering the temperance movement in its various and immediate relations to individual health and physical happiness.

One of the most important and interesting of human concerns is the enjoyment of health, inasmuch as without it all sublunary blessings would be tasteless, and life itself be irksome. The evils, however, would not rest here; for it is a well-established fact, that *health* and *virtue* are nearly as closely related as body and soul—that they flow from the same source—that our physical nature holds our moral nature, in a great measure, in dependence—that, when the habits of the *animal* economy are bad, the *moral* habits cannot be good, disease being often the parent of crime. Hence, it has been very properly asserted that "Philosophy has been in the wrong, not to descend more into the physical man; there it is that the moral man lies concealed." But notwithstanding this important bearing of health upon the affairs of body and mind—of time and eternity—it is a notorious fact that, of all others, this is a subject which has been the most neglected. Man seems desirous to know every thing and every body besides himself, though

—"all wisdom centres here."

To a great extent, we have been content to *think by proxy*, and have therefore mainly left the care of our property in the hands of the lawyer, the care of our bodies in the hands of the doctor, and the care of our souls in the hands of the parson. The result of ignorance and indifference is, we have involved ourselves in a vast amount of personal and relative suffering. But we are beginning to see, as Poor Richard says, that "Trusting too much to others' care is the ruin of many, for in the affairs of *this life* men are saved, not *by* faith, but by the *want* of it. But a man's own care is profitable; for if you would have a faithful servant, and one you like, *serve yourself*." So if you would have your property, body, and soul taken care of, DO IT YOURSELF.

HYDROPATHY FOR THE PEOPLE.

PART I.

CHAPTER I.

HEALTH AND LONGEVITY.

Mankind, like all other organic beings, ought to live according to nature's laws, without pain; and die a natural death:—i. e., without illness or suffering. But with us almost every one dies from the effects of poisonous drugs, intoxicating liquors, adulterated food, want of water, air, and exercise.—R. CLARIDGE, ESQ.

LET the reader give us his undivided attention, and bring with him an unprejudiced mind, while we take into consideration the *natural duration of human life;* and also endeavor to ascertain *whether that life ought to be spent under the influence of pain and disease.*

Our object will be to show, by the aid of Scripture, philosophy, and facts, that the opinions generally entertained on these subjects are very unsound in their character, and prejudicial in their influence.

Probably no theory can come more welcome to the human mind, than that which establishes on good ground, the hope of the enjoyment of health to "a good old age." For notwithstanding the trials, vexations, and difficulties incident to this life, the love of it generally increases with our years, and is evidently one of the *inherent* principles of our nature, which cannot be explained away by any of the subtleties of the sophist, or be overcome by any assumed dignity derived from a "false philosophy." There are many of these inextinguishable principles in our nature: such as our love of freedom—

love of country—love of home, and others; but the *love of life predominates.**—"Skin for skin, yea, all that a man hath will he give for his life."

It is an admitted fact, that disease has increased and the duration of human life decreased, from the time of the Patriarchs down to our own days, and more especially in civilized countries; but the *cause* of this fact, which does not lie very deep, we have interested ourselves very little about. At present the popular opinion is, that the natural duration of human life is seventy years; which opinion is certainly not founded upon facts or observation, for these go to prove that about one fourth of the children that are born die within the *first eleven months* of life; one third within *twenty-three months;* and one half before they reach their *eighth year.*† Two thirds of mankind die before they reach the thirty-ninth year; and three fourths before the fifty-first; so that, as Buffon observes, of *nine* children that are born, only *one* arrives at the age of seventy-three; of thirty, only *one* lives to the age of eighty; while out of 200, only one lives to the age of ninety; and in the last place, out of 11,996, only one drags on a languid existence to the age of 100 years. The mean term of life is, according to the same author, eight years in a new-born child. As the child grows older, his existence becomes more secure; and after the first year he may reasonably be expected to live to the age of thirty-three. Life becomes gradually firmer up to the age of seven; when the child, after going through the dangers of dentition, will probably live forty-two years and three months. After this period the sum of probabilities, which had gradually

* There is nothing of which men are so fond, and withal so careless, as life.—*Bruyers.*

† When we contemplate a churchyard, the earth of which is composed, in a great measure, of the bodies of infants, it is natural for us to fancy, but surely it is not reasonable for us to believe, that these beings were born for no other purpose than to die. Fault must exist some where; it cannot be in the providence of God; it must therefore attach to the improvidence and indiscretion of man. Consequences as fatal originate from ignorance as from crime.—*Reid's Essays on Insanity, etc.*

increased, undergoes a progressive decrease; so that a child of fourteen cannot be expected to live beyond thirty-seven years and five months; a man of thirty, twenty-eight years more; and in the last place, a man of eighty-four, but one year more. Such is the result of observation and of calculations on the different degrees of probabilities of human life, by Halley, Kresbroom, Wargentin, Buffon, etc., etc.

As the popular opinion cannot therefore be founded on the above, or on any well-founded statements of a similar description, we must look for its basis some where else. And it is likely we shall find it resulting from a misunderstanding of the 10th verse of the 90th Psalm, which says, "The days of our years are three-score years and ten, and if by reason of strength they be four-score years, yet is there strength, labor, and sorrow, for it is soon *cut off*, and we fly away." Let the reader observe, that rightly to understand an author, we must consider the circumstances under which he wrote, and also, if possible, the general drift of his observations and reasonings. It may, therefore, be proper to observe, that this Psalm is generally admitted to have been written by Moses, and that it has special reference to the sentence passed upon Israel in the wilderness, for their unbelief, murmuring, and rebellion against the Lord. The sentence declared that their carcasses should fall in the wilderness—that they should be wasted by a series of miseries for thirty-eight years together, until they were all destroyed; excepting Joshua and Caleb, in whom "was found another spirit, and who followed the Lord fully." Let us also carefully observe, that Moses is not speaking of the lives of men in general, but merely adverting to an *awful fact*, which was actually taking place at that time among the rebellious Israelites in the "great and terrible wilderness." That he was not speaking of the lives of men generally, may be inferred from the fact, that he, as well as many of his brethren, lived to considerably more than even ninety years. Moreover, as he complains of the people being CUT OFF through the displeasure of God, it is reasonable to suppose that he was not alluding to the period during which men were *capable* of living, but simply to the *fact*, that owing to the judgments of the Almighty, which befell the Israelites on account of their sins, but *few* of them attained a more lengthened existence than seventy or eighty years. "For we are consumed," he says, "by thine anger, and by thy wrath we are troubled."—"It is soon CUT OFF," etc.; language indicating that they died—not a *natural* death, having reached the END of the natural term of life, but were "*consumed*,"—"*cut off*."*

The eminent Dr. Farre, in his evidence before the parliamentary committee, appointed in 1843, to inquire into the causes, extent, and consequences of drunkenness, gave it as his opinion, that by the last grant of Providence to man, the natural term of his life is 120 years; in confirmation of which he quoted, Gen. vi. 3: "My spirit shall not always strive with man, for that he also is flesh; yet his days shall be an hundred and twenty years." He also further observes, "That where disease, arising from other causes, does not shorten it [human life], the reason why so few attain that age [120], is to be found in the excessive stimulation to which the mass of the community are continually subject." (See Appendix, B.) The history of mankind clearly shows that the above expressed intention of God was gradually carried into effect; the principle of vitality appearing to become weaker until the close of the era in which the postdiluvian Patriarchs flourished; when, although several centuries had elapsed since the deluge, we

* What a striking contrast does this case present to that given of the children of Israel when they left Egypt. Then it is said (Ps. cv. 37), The Lord brought them out "with silver and gold; and there was not one feeble person among the tribes." God's blessing upon their plain food and hard work had produced this—but now he is counteracting the order of nature—reversing nature's laws, in order to punish his rebellious people. There is nothing miraculous in the former case—it is the course of nature—in exact accordance with organic laws, which are God's laws; but there is in the latter, inasmuch as exercise in the open air, and even angel's food, sent direct from heaven, did not promote health—because God was consuming them.

find that 120 years was about the *average* of human existence. Abraham lived to the age of 175 years. His sons Isaac and Ishmael died, the former at the age of 180, and the latter at 137. Sarah, the only female of the ancient world of the duration of whose life we are accurately informed, lived 127 years. Jacob lived to the age of 147, and his son Joseph, although subject to all the excitement arising from the peculiarly trying circumstances in which he was placed, reached the age of 110. "The years of the life of Levi were an hundred, thirty, and seven years." Ex. vi. 16. Kohath, the second son of Levi, according to Archbishop Usher, was thirty years old when Jacob came into Egypt, and lived there 107; he therefore attained the same age as Levi, as did also his son Amram, the father of Moses. Moses lived to be 120 years old; while the sacred historian relates concerning him that "his eye was not dim, nor his natural force abated." So far, therefore, as the vital principle is concerned, he was a young man even at that advanced age, notwithstanding the harassing life he had led. Had he not shared the same fate as his brethren, in consequence of the improper spirit which he manifested at the "Waters of Meribah," he would have lived many years longer. He died, not a natural death, but was *cut off*. Joshua, who succeeded him in the government of Israel, died at the age of 100 years; and Eli, at a much later period, reached ninety-eight years, and did not then die of old age, or of disease, but was killed by a fall from his seat, on hearing that the Philistines had triumphed over the Israelites—had slain his sons Hophni and Phineas, and had taken the ark of God. Elisha, a man of great severity of manners, who despised ease and wealth, lived far above 100 years; and Simeon, a man full of hope and confidence in God, was distinguished by a life of ninety years.

That human life shall be greatly prolonged, beyond its present short limits, is one of the plain declarations of prophecy. The following is Bishop Lowth's translation of that sublime passage recorded in Isaiah lxv. 20, 23.

2

"No more shall there be an infant short-lived,
Nor an old man who hath not fulfilled his days;
For he that dieth a hundred years old shall die a boy,
And the sinner that shall die at an hundred years shall be deemed
accursed.
And they shall build houses and inhabit them;
And they shall plant vineyards, and *eat* the fruit of them;
They shall not build and another inhabit;
They shall not plant and another *eat;*
For as the days of a tree shall be the days of my people.
My chosen shall not labor in vain,
Neither shall they generate a short-lived race."

"Every one who has read the sacred original, must allow that this translation is literal;" indeed, it is generally admitted to be one of the best translations of this book: "and without staying in this place to settle the point respecting the number of years that it allots to man, it must be evident that it apportions to the inhabitants of this world a much longer period than three-score years and ten;"* though even that would be more than double the present *average* of human life in our country. Thus we think there is no ground, from Scripture, to suppose that mankind are enjoying the full term of human life. And the probability is, that the Scriptures have made known to us no specific or absolute limit to our life on earth, but that God has wisely made it dependent on the observance or non-observance of nature's laws.

* Anti-Bacchus. A cheap and first-rate work.—SNOW.

CHAPTER II.

THE PHILOSOPHY OF THE SUBJECT.

Philosophy, Wisdom, and Liberty support each other—he who *will not* reason is a *bigot*—he who *cannot* is a *fool*—and he who *dares not* is a *slave*.

SIR W. DRUMMOND.

HAVING, as we conceive, shown in the preceding chapter, from the Scripture of Divine truth, that the popular opinion, in reference to the natural duration of human life is erroneous, and believing that philosophy is always consonant with Holy Writ, we proceed to examine their joint testimony on the subject.

And here we premise, that God has evidently established a three-fold law, which must be obeyed by man, in order to his enjoyment of health and longevity. Those laws are *moral*, *mental*, and *organic*. These are the laws of God—the reflections of his holy and blessed character and perfections. It is evident that an infinitely wise and good Being must suit his laws to that which is to be governed. There must be *adaptation*. *Moral laws* are not suited to *irrational* creatures, nor *mental laws* to *material* things. Mere matter is governed entirely by organic laws—mind by intellectual laws—and moral beings by moral laws. Hence it is, that as moral agents, we are under moral laws, as accountable beings to God. These laws, by which we are to be governed, or by which we shall be judged and condemned at the last day, are revealed to us in the Scriptures; and have special reference to our conduct toward God, ourselves, and our fellow-men. And though the full amount of happiness or misery, resulting from the manner in which we observe these laws, will not be realized in this life, yet God has often made obedience to those laws a *condition* on which has rested the manner in which he has intended to deal with his rational creatures; this was more especially the case with the Jews, his ancient people. Hence we read of such *promises*, founded on such *conditions* as the following, viz.: "If ye will walk in my statutes, and keep my commandments and do them; then will I give you rain in due season, and the land shall yield her increase, and the trees of the field shall yield their fruit. And your thrashing shall reach into the vintage, and the vintage shall reach unto the sowing time,* and ye shall eat your bread to the full, and dwell in your land safely." "The inhabitant shall not say, I am sick." "And ye shall serve the Lord your God, and he shall bless thy bread and thy water, and I will take sickness away from the midst of thee." Ex. xxiii. 25.

On the other hand, God threatens them, "If ye will not hearken unto me, and will not do all these commandments; and if ye shall despise my statutes, or if your soul abhor my judgments, so that ye will not do all my commandments, but break my covenant, I also will do this unto you: I will even appoint over you, terror, consumption, and burning ague, that shall consume the eyes and cause sorrow of heart. And if ye will walk contrary unto me, and will not hearken unto me; if ye will not be reformed by me by those things, but will walk contrary unto me; then will I also walk contrary unto you, and I will punish you yet seven times more for your sins. And ye shall eat the flesh of your sons, and the flesh of your daughters.† The Lord shall make the pestilence cleave unto thee, until he have consumed thee from off the land. The Lord shall smite thee with consumption, and with fever, and with an

* "This is a nervous and beautiful promise of such entire plenty of corn and wine, that before they could have reaped and thrashed out their corn, the vintage should be ready, and before they could have pressed out their wine, it would be time to sow again. The prophet Amos, chap. ix. 13, expresses the same blessing in the same manner: The ploughman shall overtake the reaper, and the treader of grapes him who soweth seeds."—Dodd.

† This was literally fulfilled at the siege of Jerusalem. Josephus, "Wars of the Jews," book 7, chap. 2, gives us a particular instance in dreadful detail of a woman named Mary, who, in the extremity of the famine during the siege, killed her sucking child, roasted, and had eaten part of it when discovered by the soldiers! See also Jer. xix. 9.

extreme burning; with the blotch of Egypt, and with emerods, and with the scab, and with the itch, whereof thou canst not be healed." See Lev. xxvi. 14, etc., Deut. xxviii. 15, etc. These are astonishing declarations and prophecies, and though delivered more than 3000 years ago, are now fulfilling in the persons and sufferings of the Jews, affording demonstrable proof that obedience to the laws of God will secure his blessing, and that disobedience will insure his curse.

In the New Testament, all moral excellency is based on faith in God: on the belief of his paternal goodness, and the merciful and gracious character of the Lord Jesus Christ. The work of the Holy Spirit on the heart, producing repentance toward God and faith in our Lord Jesus Christ! enabling the subject of its influence to turn from sin, and to walk in the ways of God.

We are also under *mental laws,* as intellectual beings. We have capacities for knowledge, improvement, and the expansion of our intellectual powers. This capability should be cultivated; because if left to itself we can expect but little progress. We differ from animals by the reason which we exercise, and for which their instinct is a substitute; if our minds are neglected, we only show that we have a capacity for improvement, but as to the actual employment of that capacity we might almost as well be brutes. Let man be trained—his capabilities be employed—give him opportunities to unfold and improve his faculties, and he shows at once his vast superiority to all the creatures amidst which he is placed. Nay, it is almost impossible to set bounds to the extent of his powers. "Who can easily weigh the vast sense of Plato, or master the keen logic of Aristotle, or grasp the scientific research of Newton, or fathom the all-comprehending philosophy of Bacon? Cultivate the human intellect, and in the chemist's laboratory it can analyze or compound the various substances of the earth; it can resolve them into their original elements, or re-construct them into their appropriate forms. Cultivate the mind, and, by an unerring geometry, it can measure the earth, and even the heavens; with the mariner's compass, it can sail a ship to any part of the globe, and at any hour tell the place which she occupies on the immense expanse of water. Cultivate the mind, and availing itself of steam, made of nature's beverage, it can effect land or water traveling with the speed of the wind; inventing types, it can receive and communicate thought to an indefinable extent; and, by reason and memory, it can possess itself of the knowledge of all antiquity." Is not such a mind worth cultivating? Let us remember that every child has this mind in embryo! That it will be trained in some form. Reading, study, and reflection are as necessary to mental health and vigor as food, digestion, and exercise are to physical. By the diligent use of these a man may excel in intellectual things, but if he neglects them, he remains mentally sick and dwarfish.

We are also under organic laws, having organic bodies. These bodies were originally formed of the earth, and are earthy. They also require sustenance, and preservation from evil, etc. Therefore, food in proper quantity and quality, air, exercise, etc., are necessary to its well-being. Obedience to any one of these laws will not of itself secure the three-fold end. Obeying the organic and intellectual laws, and yet rebelling against the moral, may bring upon us the chastising rod of our Heavenly Father, though this mode of punishing sin is not so often adopted by Him toward us, under the Christian dispensation, as it was toward the Jews, ours being a more spiritual economy. Neglect of the organic laws will produce disease, pain, and premature death. A man may be very intellectual and devotional, but this will neither prevent disease, sustain life, nor avert other calamities. Nor is it right for a man to pray against sickness or peril, if he neglect the laws which affect the physical constitution. He would be thus tempting God to reverse the laws of the universe. This is a subject which has been much misunderstood, and has led to "charging God foolishly," with a large amount of the suffering of the world, but of which man has been the real author. We shall therefore pay a little more attention to this part of the subject, and try to "justify the ways of God to men," by throwing the blame upon its proper authors. When a man who thinks, as well as sees, suffers his eye to range over the various minor systems which compose the one great scheme of the universe; when he looks at the planetary system, and beholds worlds whirling in countless numbers, with inconceivable rapidity, yet infallible precision; when he dwells on the vegetable system, and sees myriads of plants rising from the same earth, living in the same air, warmed by the same sun, watered by the same rain, yet differing from each other, and affording year after year each his own peculiar product, with unerring exactitude; when, with more inquisitive glance, he penetrates the thicker veil with which nature has sustained the chemical world, and watches the several phenomena resulting from chemical operations—combustion, putrefaction, vegetation, fermentation, etc.—observes the unfailing exactitude with which all these render obedient homage to the one great law of affinity; then, when he looks inward and contemplates his own system, beautiful as the most beautiful, and not less worthy of omnipotent wisdom than the most worthy; when he looks inward, and beholds there all confusion and imperfection; when he perceives that, of all the systems of nature, that of man alone is liable to derangement, etc.;—the mind cannot but be irresistibly struck with the anomaly, and the tongue cannot but exclaim, "Why is it so?" It is thus: that while all other systems of the universe are sustained and governed by immutable laws, as gravitation, chemical affinity, instinct, etc., etc., the system of man depends solely for support upon laws, the perfect or imperfect fulfillment of which has been left dependent on the capricious conduct of man himself. I am not attempting to prove that man is not "born to die;" I am only endeavoring to show that he was not, by God, subject to disease, and premature death. I cannot believe that it formed a part of the original design of the Almighty Architect of the universe, that one half of mankind should die before they have attained the age of eight years; that is, before they have lived long enough to fulfill any one conceivable intention; in fact, before they are themselves fully formed. If any man dies while any one of his organs is unimpaired, he dies prematurely, and before he has fulfilled the final cause of his existence. For God is an economist in every thing; he creates nothing in vain—never falls short, or exceeds the object in view. There is but one legitimate cause of death; and that is *old age.* And here we see the goodness of God: there is nothing painful in death from old age, if the soul has found peace with God, through our Lord Jesus Christ. It makes its advances with a gradual and steady step, which is scarcely noted; and the old man drops into the tomb almost insensibly—"his end is peace." Thus it will appear that nature's laws are immutable, and unchangeable, and that when they are obeyed there will be no exception to the enjoyment of health and longevity. Many such instances have occurred since the Christian era—a proof that man is not so constituted as to render it inevitable that he should live in a state of disease, and die at so early a period as now bounds his existence. Combe, in his highly talented work, the "Constitution of Man, considered in relation to external objects,"* says, "I hope I do not err in stating that neither disease nor death, in early or middle life, can take place under the ordinary administration of Providence, except when the organic laws have been infringed." The pains of premature death, then, are the punishments of infringement of these laws; and the object of that chastisement probably is, to impress upon us the necessity of obeying them, that we may live, and to prevent our abusing the remedial process inherent to a great extent in our constitution. That death in old age only is the natural institution of the creation, is evident from all the philosophic reasoning we can bring to bear upon the subject. Drs. Smith and Arnott, in their celebrated report to the government, in 1835, say, "There is nothing in the physiologi-

* Published by Fowlers & Wells, New York.

cal constitution of man to prevent his long surviving the age of seventy years, or more, if the causes which now prevent their doing so were removed." Dr. S. Graham, in his excellent "Lectures to Young Men," observes, "If mankind always lived precisely as they ought to live, they would, as a general rule, most certainly pass through the several states of life, from infancy to old age, without sickness; enjoying, through their long-protracted years, health, serenity, and peace; individual and social happiness; and gradually wear out their vital energies, and finally lie down, and fall asleep in death, without agony—without pain." Disease is not natural, but artificial; as much so as any production can be artificial. Man, at his creation, was endowed with the gift of health, and was destined to enjoy longevity, and not to be the sickly, suffering creature we now behold him. "He was designed to enjoy health, and sink by slow degrees into the bosom of his parent earth, without disease or pain."—*Vegetable Regimen.* Hesiod tells us that "before the time of Prometheus,* mankind were exempt from all suffering; and that death, when at length it came, approached like sleep, and gently closed their eyes." And Dr. Campbell speaks with his accustomed force and perspicuity, when, in the first number of that prodigy, the *Christian Witness* (which has obtained a circulation of thirty thousand per month), he gives it as his opinion that "premature decay, sickness, and death are matters very much under the control of man." Dr. Bigel asserts, "Man is, physically and morally, the author of his own ills." If we lived on healthy food and drink, such a thing as disease would be impossible.—*Whitlaw.*

Captain Claridge has presented his readers with some very striking remarks on man's organism, in which he clearly shows that man, as an organized being, must be subject to the organic laws. An organized being is one which derives its ex-

* Prometheus first instructed mankind in the culinary and other uses of fire, and also set them the example of slaughtering an ox.

istence from a previously existing organized being, which subsists on food, which grows, decays, and dies. The first law, then, that must be obeyed, in order to render an organized being perfect in its kind, is that the germ from whence it springs shall be complete in all its parts, and sound in its whole constitution. If we sow an acorn in which some vital part has been destroyed altogether, the seedling plant, and the full-grown oak (if ever it attain maturity), will be deficient in the lineaments which are wanting in the embryo root; if we sow an acorn, entire in its parts, but only half ripened, or damaged in its whole texture by damp or other causes, the seedling oak will be feeble, and will probably die early. A similar law holds good in regard to man. For instance, a man, from high living and indolence, contracts gout; his sons, however temperate, may nevertheless be afflicted with gout by inheritance; that is, supposing gout to be an hereditary disease, as some assert. Here we have a clue to that declaration of Jehovah, in which he declares he "will visit the iniquity of the fathers upon the children," which he does sometimes "upon the children's children, unto the third and fourth generation."

A second organic law, according to Mr. Claridge, is, that the organized being, the moment it is ushered into life, and as long as it continues to live, must be supplied with food, light, air, and every other physical element requisite for its support, in due quantity, and of the kind best suited to its peculiar constitution. Obedience to this law is rewarded with a vigorous and healthy development of its powers; and in animals, with a pleasing consciousness of existence, and aptitude for the performance of their natural functions. Disobedience is punished with feebleness, stunted growth, general imperfections, or an early death. A few facts shall illustrate this. At a meeting of the "British Association," held in Edinburgh, in 1834, there was read an abstract, by Dr. J. Clarke, of a registry kept in the Lying-in Hospital of Great Britain-st., Dublin, from the year 1758 to the end of 1833, from which it appeared that, in 1781, when the hospital was imperfectly ventilated, every sixth child died, within nine days of its birth, of convulsive disease; and that after means of thorough ventilation had been adopted, the mortality of infants within the same time, in five succeeding years, was reduced to nearly one in twenty; thus showing that, as they approached to perfect obedience of organic laws, human life was preserved. Again, the Society of Friends, who are composed of all ranks and classes, and whose pursuits are as various as their local habitations, and who are therefore equally subject to all the ordinary contingencies of life, are nevertheless remarkable for their temperance, health, and longevity. An inquiry having been made some years ago, previously to the formation of an assurance society exclusively for themselves, a search was made into the public register of the parish of Chesterfield, in Derbyshire, and also that of Chesterfield Monthly Meeting of Friends. The following are the results: the united ages of one hundred individuals, successively buried in Chesterfield churchyard, ending November 16, 1834, were 2515 years and six months—making the average of each life twenty-five years and two months. But of the individuals buried among "Friends," ending the 27th of November, 1834, the total of their ages were 4790 years and seven months—giving an average of forty-seven years and ten months, or nearly double that of the general population. Pursuing the calculation still further, they found that only two of the one hundred buried in the churchyard reached eighty and upward; but among Friends, nineteen attained to eighty or more. In the churchyard, twelve of the number were buried whose ages were seventy and upward; but of Friends, thirty died who were at least seventy years old.* These facts speak volumes

* From their *Annual Monitor*, for 1836, it appears that rather more than two hundred adults are recorded, of whom ninety were from sev enty to eighty-four years old, averaging full eighty years each; and of these one fourth were from seventy-eight to ninety-eight, and ten produce an average of full ninety-four years. Now it should be remembered that these statistics were obtained and published by the above respectable society, in connection with the question of assurance, and that alone.

in favor of our system; and whenever our principles are more generally adopted by that religious society, as we believe they will be, not only by them, but also by all thinking, independent people, there is no question but their difference of health and longevity will be still more striking.

The effect of intemperance in shortening life is strikingly exemplified in the contrast afforded by other classes of society with the Friends. For it appears from accurate calculation that in London, only one in forty attains the age of eighty, while among the Friends not less than one in ten reaches that age.*

A *third organic law*, applicable to man, as stated by Mr. Claridge, is, that he shall duly exercise his organs, this condition being an indispensable prerequisite of health. The reward of obedience to this law, is enjoyment in the very act of exercising the functions, a pleasing consciousness of existence, and the acquisition of numberless gratifications of which labor, or the exercise of our powers, is the procuring means. Disobedience is punished with derangement and sluggishness of the functions, with general uneasiness or positive pain, and the denial of gratification to numerous faculties.

Health and longevity, in the wide and physiological acceptation, consist in all the actions of which living beings are capable, not only the internal action, as of the heart, vessels, etc., but also of the external action of the limbs, in running, leaping, etc. All physiologists agree that life consists in the constant wasting and reproduction of the body, particle by particle, by a

where it became their interest not to exaggerate; and they are the more valuable to us as being incidental.

* Dr. Macnish says the children of drunkards "are more than ordinarily liable to inherit all the diseases of those from whom they are sprung." On this account the chances of long life are much diminished among the children of drunkards. In proof of this it is only necessary to remark that, according to the London bills of mortality, one half of the children born in the metropolis die before attaining their third year; while of the children of Friends, one half actually attain the age of forty-seven years.

perpetual pulling down of the old materials, and a perpetual replacement of them by new; by perpetual disorganization, and perpetual reorganization. The first process therefore is, What? Eating? No: it is the wasting, the pulling down. You must waste before you can nourish it. Does not the appetite precede the act of eating? And what is appetite but a sensation that the body has suffered waste, and calling upon us to repair it? The natural means by which the body is disorganized are, the exhalations from the lungs, of the several secretions required for the assimilation of our food, as the gastric juice, bile, etc. The natural law, therefore, appears to be, that every one who desires to enjoy the pleasures of health must expend in labor the energy which the Creator has infused into his limbs, which he may do in various ways. The penalty for neglecting this law of nature is imperfect digestion and disturbed sleep; debility of body and mental lassitude; and if carried to a certain length, confirmed bad health and early death. Thus thousands are daily tampering with their health; aggravating human depravity; creating or increasing disease; and then, laying the blame to Providence, they malign the character of the ever-blessed God. He merely maintains the law of his throne, that *cause* (the violation of his laws) shall produce *effect* (disease and early death). As society has not obeyed this law, the consequences are, the higher orders despise labor, and suffer as above; and the lower orders are oppressed with harder living, and more work than their masters' horses, etc., and hence suffer exhaustion; a desire is created for stimulants, such as alcoholic drinks, tea, spices, etc., which produce disease and shorten life. In this we discover the chief sources of disease and premature death. In this we discover also the chief sources of the enormous inequality of the distribution of property—one living, a mass of bloated disease, on, perhaps, £300,000 per annum, while another is doomed to a life of squalid misery, and drags out a wretched existence on some few pounds. And yet we are told these things are *ordained* by a merciful Providence! Impossible! Believe it who can; I will not try!* Why not? Because God never could design that his creatures should live a short and miserable life, and then die a violent and unnatural death. The above evils produce these effects, and lead to this result; therefore, they are not of divine appointment. To say they are, is a reflection upon the Deity, of which no rightly constituted mind will be guilty. God is always consistent with himself; his laws, physical and moral, do not clash. There is a glorious uniformity in all his works and ways; and all his truths are as connected as an undivided chain. But there seems to be a sort of consolation in being able to saddle the blame of any wrong course we have taken upon others—after the example of Adam and Eve. Hence, if the lady cannot please herself with the goods sent home, she visits the shopkeeper with a gentle scolding, and returns the articles upon his hands; the shopkeeper is vexed, reprimands the journeyman, and mulcts him in his wages; the poor journeyman is enraged, and flies, perhaps, to exciting liquors, goes home and plays the *hero* over his wife, or boxes the ears of the errand boy, who, aroused in his turn, has no resource than to kick the dog, or worry some less valiant animal. It is just the same in the political and social world. The executive is blamed, taxes are heavy, there is too much monopoly, etc., all of which are true; but the parties forget that "true genius rises above circumstances." There are some awkward things, for which we can blame neither the government nor society at large, nor any individual in it, except ourselves; this we are anxious to avoid, therefore we attribute it to Providence. If parents are afflicted with disease, it is a visitation of Providence; if they have a long train of children wailing under scrofula, blindness, etc., it is quite orthodoxly and complacently set down to the account of Providence; and on they proceed, in

* Is there not more propriety in the noble sentiment of Rumbold: "The Creator does not intend that the greater part of mankind should come into the world with saddles upon their backs, and bridles in their mouths, and a few, ready booted and spurred, to ride the rest to death."

self-congratulation, filling the world with such objects, asserting that there is no help for it—such being the will of Providence. What but ignorance and superstition* could have produced such unphilosophic and God-dishonoring views? Surely it ought never to be thought, that while wild animals, who live according to nature in obedience to organic laws, are free from contagious distempers and premature decay, an exception has been made with regard to man, the masterpiece of Creative goodness. And we never hear of their lying dead in numbers through the fields. Nor is there any reason to believe they are subject to debility, except the failure of strength consequent on their having reached the period of existence appointed to their kind by the Creator. And if we reason analogically, and consider how definitive nature is in her operations—with how much exactness she apportions the substance which forms the bones, muscles, hair, nails, etc., it can hardly be denied that the astonishing deviation from such laws, of which human disease is an instance, must be attributed to some extraneous cause acting powerfully in contravention of the order of nature. If a man rises at a late hour in the morning, with a brain-hammering headache, he soon consciously refers it to the previous night's excess either in eating or drinking, or both; and knows it is a natural consequence of his own error; yet it is as much the work of Providence as blindness in a new-born child. Nay, further; if the result of a public dinner is only indigestion, or a headache, it is a natural consequence, but if the victim of sensuality drops down dead in the street, or more quietly dies in his bed during the night, then it is a

* Thunder and lightning were considered for many ages in the same light as diseases have hitherto been, as awful visitations of Providence. In all such storms, the Deity was believed to be personally present, and to wield the thunderbolt with his "red right arm;" but science has at length shed her influence over mankind, and has consigned this creed to poetry and superstition. Let Christians, especially, beware how they commit themselves in this matter, lest they fill the mouths of infidels, and expose their own ignorance of God's laws, and arraign his wisdom and goodness.

visitation of Providence, and the coroner's jury gives a verdict accordingly. The undertaker's fees being paid, and other accounts settled, without one useful lesson, on they go again, to open a new case, like spendthrifts of life, regardless of the reducing store, saying, "To-morrow shall be as to-day, and much more abundant." We will not characterize such mental and moral delinquency by any hard names, but it does appear to us, that men have frequently been denounced and punished for opinions much less dishonorable to God, and less detrimental to human happiness.

From the whole, then, there resulteth this general conclusion: that man is an organized being; subjected to organic laws; that there is no such thing as perfect health where those laws are not obeyed; that it would be contrary to the scheme of man's existence; that the philosophy of life and health, the light of science, the testimony of all ages, and the force of argument prove it to be impossible. On the other hand, we maintain that there is nothing unreasonable in supposing it possible, with respect to the organization and vital force of man, that the one may endure and the other act, during 150 or even 200 years. One fact which gives weight to this theory, is the connection which is known to exist between the period for arriving at maturity, and the duration of human life. This deduction is based upon the principle that animals, in general, live eight times as long as they are in growing to maturity. The elephant and camel are, perhaps, among the longest livers; the former often attains to 100 years, and arrives at maturity about the twelfth year; the latter lives from seventy to ninety, and arrives at maturity about the ninth year. The horse, the mule, and the ass seldom live more than forty years, and arrive at maturity about the fifth year. They may, however, ascribe their short life, in some degree, to the improper and unnatural manner in which they are treated by man.* Thus, in an ordinary state, i. e., when

* There can be no doubt that the domestication of animals entails

nature is not forced on by art, man requires twenty-five years to attain to maturity, which would, according to the above reasoning, assign to him a life of 200 years; whereas, all that we contend for is, that "his days shall be an hundred and twenty years."

upon them many disorders and much misery. It is not uncommon for a gentleman who has three or four saddle horses in his stable, to be unable on the same day to ride one of them. An English horse, indeed, is becoming so precarious a possession, that wherever he goes it requires an English groom to keep him alive. We learn from veterinary writers, that horses are more exposed to tetanus than the human subject; that rheumatism is frequent among them, and that they are not even exempt from gout. How different this from the state of the horse in his wild state. While yet unsubdued; yet untouched by the withering hand of man, we find the animal so active and powerful, that he easily defends himself against the strongest bull. At thirty years old, and even at forty, he is known still to enjoy his full vigor.—See Newton's "Return to Nature," a good but dear work.

CHAPTER III.

FACTS AND FIGURES.

Since the mighty mind of *Bacon* beat down hypothesis, and introduced the inductive system, philosophy has reasoned from *facts;* and experimental philosophy has been applauded.—JAY.

The most perfect system has ever been allowed to be that which can reconcile and bring together the greatest number of *facts*, that come within the sphere of the subject of it. In this consists the sole glory of Newton, whose discovery rests upon no higher order of proof. Human authority seldom settles any thing with me; for whenever I have had an interest in knowing the truth, I have generally appealed from the decrees of that unsatisfactory court to the less fallible decision of the *court of fact.*—DR. DICKSON.

Facts are the arguments of God—the outworkings of his power. He who fights against *facts*, fights against God.—DR. F. LEES, F.S.A.

DR. HUFELAND, in his *Macrobitic*, a work which has been translated into nearly all European languages, after citing numerous cases of extreme longevity, says, "We ought to have some fixed ideas as to what ought to be the true term of life; but we can hardly imagine to what an extent doctors differ on this point. Some assign to man extreme longevity, while others cut life very short. We might be tempted to believe that death occasioned by old age was the true term of man's life; but a calculation established upon such a basis, would lead us into great errors, in an artificial state like ours." And this, in fact, is the very error into which people have fallen.

The learned Lichtenberg declared that the secret had been discovered of inoculating people with old age before their time; and added, "We see, every day, men thirty or forty years old, presenting all the appearance of decrepitude, deformity, wrinkles, gray hairs, and other defects, which one only expects to find in men of eighty or ninety years of age." To the inquiry, "How long, in general, can man live?" *facts* answer, "from one hundred and fifty to one hundred and seventy, and even two hundred years."

Haller, who collected most of the cases of longevity known in Europe in his time, gave examples of more than one thousand persons who attained to 100, and 110 years; sixty persons from 110 to 120; twenty-nine from 120 to 130; fifteen from 133 to 140; six from 140 to 150; and one to 169 years. From the statistics of Russia, it appears that, in 1830, there were in that country, among others, the following instances of longevity: one hundred and twenty persons who had reached from 116 to 120 years; one hundred and twenty-one from 120 to 125; three from 125 to 130; five from 130 to 140; one to 145; three from 150 to 155; one to 160; and one to 165. In the tables of mortality for England and Wales, commencing at 1813, and ending with 1830, being a period of eighteen years, we find that from the age of eighty-one to that of one hundred and twenty-four, upward of 245,000 persons were buried, of whom more than seven hundred exceeded one hundred years.

The following, with some additions, are copied from Baker's "Curse of Britain:"

William Dupe,	95
His father,	102
His grandfather,	108
Michell Vivian,	100
John Crossley,	100
Lewis Cornaro,	100
Admiral H. Rolvenden,	100
Jane Milner,	102
Eleanor Aymer,	103
Eleanor Pritchard,	103
Her sisters, who are still living,	104 108
William Popman,	103
William Marmon,	103
Wife of Cicero,	103
Stender,	103

Epimenides,	157
Robert Lynch,	160
Letitia Cox,	160
Joice Heath,	162
Sarah Rovin,	164
William Edwards,	168
Henry Jenkins,	169
John Rovin,	172
Peter Porton,	185
Mongate,	185
Petratsch Czarten,	185
Thomas Cam,	207
Numas de Cugna,	370

In giving a more detailed account of individuals in different ages and countries, who have been remarkable for health and longevity, we may mention Democrates, the searcher of nature, a man of good temper and serene mind, who lived in good health to one hundred and nine years. Zeno, the founder of the Stoical sect, and a master of the art of self-denial, attained nearly to the age of one hundred years. Palemon, of Athens, in his youth led a life of debauchery and drunkenness; but when about thirty years of age, he entered the school of Zenocrates, when in a state of intoxication: he was so struck with the eloquence of the Academician, and the force of his arguments, that from that time he renounced his dissipated habits, and adopted the principles of the "Nature's Beverage Society"—drinking no other beverage than water. He died at an extreme old age.—*See Tem. Biblioth. Class in loco.* Cato, who was said to have had "an iron body, and an iron mind," was fond of a country life, a great enemy to physicians, and lived to near one hundred years.

A very remarkable collection, in regard to the duration of human life, in the time of Vespasian, has been presented to us by Pliny, from the records of the census, a source worthy of great credit. It there appears that, in the year when that numbering took place, the seventy-sixth of our era, there were living in that part of Italy which lies between the Apennines and the Po only, 124 men who had attained to the age of 100 years and upward, viz.: fifty-one of 100; fifty-seven of 110; two of 125; four of 130; four of from 132 to 137; and three of 140. Besides these, there were living in Parma, five men, three of whom were 120, and two were 130; in Placentia, one of 130; at Facentia, a woman of 132; and in Velligacian, a small town near Placentia, there were living ten persons, six of whom were 110, and four were 120.

Francis Secardia Hongo died A.D. 1702, aged 114 years, ten months, and twelve days. He left behind him forty-nine children—was never sick in his life. His sight, hearing, memory, and agility were the surprise of all who knew him. At 110, he lost all his teeth; but he cut two large ones, in his upper jaw, the year before he died. He never used to drink strong drinks, coffee, etc.; never used tobacco; and his only drink was water. His habits, in other respects, were temperate.

In the "Miscellanea Curiosa" may be found an interesting account of a man 120 years of age, without the loss of a tooth, and of a brisk and lively disposition, whose only drink, from his infancy, was pure water.

Sinclair, in his "Code of Health, etc.," speaks of the famous civilian, Andrew Tieraqueaus, who is said, for thirty years together, to have given yearly a book, and by the same wife a son, to the world, and who lived to a good old age. He never drank any thing but water, from his infancy.

In the year 1792, died in the duchy of Holstein, an industrious day-laborer, named Stender, in the 103d year of his age. His food, for the most part, was oatmeal and buttermilk. He rarely ever ate flesh; he was never sick, and could not be put out of temper. He had the greatest trust in Providence; his chief dependence was in the goodness of God, which no doubt greatly conduced to his health and longevity.

Ant. Senish, a farmer of Puy, in Limoges, died in 1770, in

the 111th year of his age. He labored till within fourteen days of his death. His teeth and hair remained, and his sight had not failed him. His usual food was chestnuts and turkey-corn. He had never been bled, nor used any medicine.

Died, on the 26th of June, 1838, at Bybrook, Mrs. Letitia Cox, upward of 160 years of age. She declared she had never drank any thing but water during the whole of her life; as did also another woman, at Holland Estate, who died eighteen months before, at the age of 140.

Lewis Cornaro, a Venetian nobleman, died at Padua, in 1565, at above 100 years of age. In early life he had been very intemperate, and consequently greatly diseased. From his thirty-fifth to his fortieth year, his life was a burden to him. By a regular way of living, he repaired his health, in a remarkable manner; and in his eighty-first year says, "I am free from apprehension of disease, because I have nothing in my constitution for a disease to feed upon—from the apprehension of death, because I have spent a life of reason. I know that, barring accidents, no violent disease can touch me. I must be dissolved by a gentle and gradual decay, like oil in a lamp, which affords no longer life to the dying taper. But such a death cannot happen of a sudden."

Richard Lloyd died near Montgomery, aged 132 years and ten months. He was a tall, strong, upright man; had no gray hairs; had lost none of his teeth; and could see to read without spectacles. His food was bread, cheese, and butter, for the most part; and his drink whey, buttermilk, or water, and nothing else. But being persuaded by a neighboring gentleman to eat flesh-meat, and drink malt liquor, he soon fell off, and died.

Dr. Lower speaks of a man in the north, aged 120, who had been accustomed to eat very little animal food, but lived upon oatmeal pottage and potatoes, and sometimes he took a little milk. He was a laboring man, and never remembered being sick.

Dr. E. Baynard gives an account of one Seth Unthank, then

(1706) living at Bath, whose chief drink was sour buttermilk. He was wonderfully nimble, and, not above two years before, had walked from Bath to London, 106 miles, in two days, and came home again in two days more. His uncle was 126 years old when he died, and had been one of the Bishop of Durham's pensioners. The doctor also speaks of one John Bailes, of Northampton, whom he visited, then living, in his 129th year. He says he had a very strong voice, and spake very loud; and told the doctor he had buried the whole town (except three or four) twenty times over. "Strong drink," quoth the old man, "kills 'em all." He was never drunk; his drink was water, small beer, and milk; and his food, for the most part, was brown bread* and cheese. He cared not much for flesh-meats.

Mrs. Hudson lived 105 years, and then died of an acute disease, brought on by catching cold. She could see to thread a needle at that age. Her food was very little else than bread and milk, all her lifetime.

Louis Wholeham, of Ballinamona, Cork, died at the age of 118 years and seven months. He had not lost a tooth, nor had he one gray hair on his head. His diet, all through life, was mostly potatoes and milk;† but, on an average, he had

* Bread being an article so much in use, it is of importance we should use the best—that which is most calculated to promote health. The best bread is made of equal parts of wheat and rye, ground down together, no bran being taken out, and made into unfermented biscuits. Fine wheat flour, being of a starchy nature, is apt to occasion constipation, acidity, and flatulence. This bread would be found of great service to weak stomachs, which are often injured by the least extrication of air, when bread ferments a second time in the stomach.

† Much has been said for and against milk. In favor of it, we are told of persons being cured of long-standing diseases, by living exclusively upon it, for six or seven years; and also we are referred to the health and longevity of some who have made much use of it. (See Appendix, C.) On the other hand, we are told that the cows about our towns and cities are greatly diseased, in consequence of being subjected to the unnatural and unhealthy influences of bad air, want of exercise, and improper food. Cows are also diseased, we are told, through the vegeta-

flesh one day in the week, until the last ten years, when he took a dislike to it, and could not eat it. It is a remarkable fact, showing how we cling to life, that he declared, on his death-bed, that he should have been more resigned to die eighty years ago than he was at that time.

Joice Heath, of America, was being exhibited in several of their large towns, at the age of 162; and when asked what was her food, said, "Corn-bread and potatoes is what I eat."

Francisco Lupatsoli, of Smyrna, lived 113 years. He drank nothing but water and milk; having used neither tea, coffee, etc. He lived chiefly upon bread, figs, etc. He could hear well, and see without spectacles, even to the last.

Zeno is said to have died at the age of ninety-eight years, having never experienced any sickness or indisposition whatever.

If we refer to the American Indians, we find, at the first arrival of Europeans among them, it was not uncommon to find persons who were above 100 years old. They lived frugally, and drank only pure water. Strong drinks were unknown to them till introduced by Christians, by whom they have been taught to drink; and now they hardly reach half the age of their parents.—*Kalm.*

The same traveler says the natives of Shetland give an account of one Fairville, who arrived at the age of 102, and never drank any malt liquor, distilled water, or wine. They say his son lived longer than he; that his grandchildren lived to a great age, and seldom or never drank any stronger liquor than milk, or water, or bland. This last is made of buttermilk, mixed with water.

The natives of Sierra Leone, whose climate is said to be the worst on earth, are very temperate; they subsist entirely on

bles they eat; and that, if the animal be diseased, so must the milk, as also the butter and cheese. (See Whitlaw's "Treatise on Fever," and Clark's "Treatise on Pulmonary Consumption.") Annatto and arsenic are sometimes added to cheese; the former to give it color, and the latter freshness and tenderness. (See "Library of Health," vol. ii. p. 9.)

small quantities of boiled rice, with occasional supplies of fruit, and drink only cold water ; in consequence of which they are strong and healthy, and live as long as men in the most propitious climates.

Herodotus tells us that the average life of the Macrobians was 120 years, and that they never drank any thing stronger than milk. But if there be one portion of the globe more than another, to which the general consent of mankind accords the first place in point of beauty and symmetry, it will be the Circassian race; and we are much gratified in being able to adduce this nation as an illustration of the position we have taken. We will make one short extract from "Travels in Circassia, Kirm, etc.," by E. Spencer, Esq., who says, "Owing to the robust firmness and temperate manner of living, the Circassians generally attain an advanced age; their diseases being neither numerous nor dangerous." This must be attributed, independently of their simple diet, to their constant exercise, pure air, etc.

It is mentioned in Keppis' "Life of Captain Cook," that when that great navigator first visited the New Zealanders he was astonished at the perfect and uninterrupted health they were found to enjoy. In all the visits which were paid to this people, not a single person was found who appeared to have any complaint, nor among the number who were seen naked, was once perceived the slightest eruption on the skin, or the least mark which indicated that such eruption had formerly existed. "Their wounds heal with remarkable facility, without any applications. It abounds with a great number of old men, many of whom, by the loss of their teeth and hair, appeared to be very ancient, and yet none of them were decrepit. Although they are not equal to the young in muscular strength, they do not come behind them with regard to cheerfulness and vivacity. Water, as far as our navigators could discover, is the universal and daily liquor of the New Zealanders."*

* How are the mighty fallen! In the South Seas, and also in New Zealand, the most heart-rending contrast is now presented to their former

But we may refer to our own country for facts and illustrations equally striking. In the "Patriot," of the 12th of October, are notices of the death of four individuals then recently deceased; of whom one was in his ninety-second year, another in his ninety-fifth, a third in his 100th, and the other in his 114th. Also in the said paper of December 4th, 1843, is recorded the death of Jane Milner, in her 102nd year. She was a member of the Moravian Church, at Baildon.

William Dupe died at Oxford, September 23rd, 1843, aged ninety-five years. His eldest surviving child is sixty years of age; the youngest, an infant of two years old. Up to a very recent period, he exhibited no marked appearance of either mental or bodily decay; and at Christmas last (1842), he addressed a large meeting at a temperance festival. The most remarkable facts in connection with the long life and great vigor of this patriarch is, that he was the son and grandson of water drinkers. The united ages of these three persons exceed three centuries; the grandfather attaining 108 years; the father 102. Two facts, exhibiting the strength and consistency

comparative state of health and happiness. Disease and mortality abound almost unparalleled in character, arising from the introduction of strong drinks. Traders from Christian countries threaten to depopulate these islands in a very few years, unless missionary influence and exertions, in connection with teetotalism, prevent it, and save them from their fate. That we do not exaggerate, we refer our readers to the state of the population when Captain Cook landed, and their present state—the contrast is humiliating and alarming. Then, according to the statements of A. Chapin, M.D., late a resident in those islands, the population was not less than 400,000. Estimating a period of fifty-seven years since their discovery by Europeans, and also taking into account losses occasioned by their wars, he supposes, with great reason, that their population should have increased at least one half, making at present a probable total of 600,000. The terrible facts, however, are well known, that the population of these islands only amounts to 135,000, making the fearful loss, during fifty-seven years, of not less than 465,000, which, Mr. C. adds, is chargeable to the customs or vices carried there from other places. These appalling facts will excite less surprise, when it is known, on the authority of Mr. Ellis, that a sum of not less than 12,000 dollars was expended in Tahite alone, in one year, for intoxicating drinks.

of William Dupe's attachment to water are recorded. When a young man he was most rudely threatened with strong drink by compulsion; he at length defended himself by a blow which broke his assailant's jaw-bone. When the lamp of life was flickering, he steadfastly refused to take wine, ordered by his medical attendant, and even made it one of his last requests, that there should be no drinking at his funeral.

John Crossley, Esq., whose food in the latter part of his life was chiefly milk, lived above 100 years.

Helen Grey died in her 105th year. She was of small stature, exceedingly lively, peaceable, and good-tempered; and a few years before her death she acquired new teeth.

Thomas Garrick, of the county of Fife, in the 108th year of his age, was in the possession of great vigor; he died on the 3rd of July, 1847, being then 151 years of age. For twenty years previous he had never been confined to his bed by sickness.

Ann Parker, who was the oldest woman in Kent, died at 109. Another old woman died recently in the western part of England, at the age of 110, leaving 450 descendants, more than 200 of whom attended her funeral. Also a Scotch newspaper, published in 1839, notices an old woman, then living in Glasgow, who was 130 years of age, and who, for the last fifty years, had not taken intoxicating drinks. She had never any occasion to take drugs, nor was a lancet ever applied to her frame. She was perfectly free from affections of the chest, and during the last century had been a perfect stranger to pain. Her pulse did not exceed seventy strokes per minute. Her grandfather died at the age of 129; her father at 120. Her grandfather and father were both very temperate.

In the year 1757, J. Effingham died in Cornwall, in the 144th year of his age. He never drank strong heating liquors, seldom eat flesh, and always lived remarkably temperate. Till his 100th year he scarcely knew what sickness was; and eight days before his death he walked three miles.

The Countess of Desmond lived to the age of 145, and preserved her faculties nearly to the last. Upon the ruin of the house of Desmond, she was obliged, at the age of 140, to travel to London from Bristol, to solicit relief from the court, being reduced to poverty. Lord Bacon says she renewed her teeth twice or thrice.

Thomas Parr, of Shropshire, maintained himself by day labor, which it would be much better for those to be employed in who are injuring the public by selling what they call *Parr's Life Pills*, but which, like most others, are *Death Pills.* When about 120, he married a widow for his second wife. Till his 130th year he performed his usual work, and was accustomed to thrash. Some years before his death his eyes and memory began to fail; but his hearing and senses continued sound to the last. In his 152nd year he was taken to court, where he only lived nine months, in consequence of the change in his mode of living. When his body was opened by Dr. Harvey, his bowels were found to be in the most perfect state. He died merely of a plethora, occasioned by living too high. Parr's great-grandson died at Cork a few years ago, at the age of 103.

Several of the above cases show that a good constitution, so favorable to longevity, may transmit a good *stamen vita;* and this confirms our observations on the first organic law.

On a long freestone slab, in Cairy Church, near Cardiff, is the following inscription: "Here lieth the body of William Edwards, of the Cairy, who departed this life the 24th of February, A.D. 1688. Anno Que statis suæ 168."

In the year 1670 died Henry Jenkins, aged 169. His monument is in the church of Bolton-upon-Swale, in Yorkshire It was proved from the registers in chancery, and other courts, that he had appeared 140 years before as an evidence, and had an oath administered to him. When he was above the age of 100 he could swim across rapid rivers.

The last case we shall cite is that recorded in the "County Chronicle," of December 13th, 1791; in which it is stated that "Thomas Cam, according to the parish register of St. Leonard, Shoreditch, died the 28th of January, 1588, aged 207 years!"

The correspondent of that paper adds, "This is an instance of longevity so far exceeding any other on record, that one is disposed to suspect some mistake, either in the register or in the extract." But on application to the proper authorities he received the following:

> 1588. BURIALLES. Fol: 35
>
> Thomas Cam was buriel ye 22 inst of Januarye Aged 207 years.
>
> Holywell Street.
>
> Geo. Garrow
>
> Copy August 25, 1832. Parish Clerk.

"It thus appears," adds our correspondent, "that Cam was born in the year 1381, in the fourth of Richard II., living through the reign of that monarch, and through those of the whole of the following sovereigns, viz.: Henry IV., Henry V., Henry VI., Edward IV., Edward V., Richard III., Henry VII., Henry VIII., Edward VI., Mary, and to the thirteenth of Elizabeth."

It has also been justly observed, that wild animals do not live a life of misery and pain, nor, except by accident, do they die young. And we ask, why should man? unless by artificial means, and a departure from nature's laws, he injures and destroys himself. Of all animals, he is not only the handsomest, but the strongest, according to his weight. No animal, not even the lion, has such firmly-knitted joints, such strong muscles, or such a well-built frame as man. No other animal has calves to his legs; and if the joints of the whole body be taken into consideration, those of man will be found far superior to those of other animals. Few animals can equal man in supporting long trials of strength, and enduring fatigue. The strongest horse, or dog, cannot bear the fatigue of walking so long as man. We have examples of savages passing three days and nights without repose or nourishment, at the same time marching quickly through their native wilds, pursuing or pursued, when even their horses and dogs were wearied and left behind. Thus we see, notwithstanding our frequent violations of organic laws, how much we are capable of doing or suffering. No animal can support changes of climate like man: witness the Norwegian, wending his way through the Arabian deserts, where the traces of none, save the tiger's foot, are seen. We have numerous examples, too, of men subduing wild animals, by the main strength of their muscles and joints. These facts admitted, and they cannot be denied, is it not evident that man, who in his wild state is capable of doing and suffering so much, has in his civilized state greatly infringed the organic laws, and is suffering the consequence, in an emaciated frame, a short life of disease and suffering, and an early and agonizing death. How often do the votaries of intemperate indulgence say, "A short life and a merry one." The former they effectually secure; but their very indulgences deprive them of the latter.

Some suppose climate has every thing to do with health and longevity. That it has something, we readily admit; but it has not so much as many are disposed to believe. There can, however, be no doubt that Sweden, Norway, Denmark, and England have, in modern times, furnished the greatest number of old men, as will be seen by the list we have presented. Dr. Cheyne says there is no place in the world more likely to lengthen out life than England, especially those parts of it that have a free, open air, and a gravelly and chalky soil, if, to due exercise and abstemiousness, a plain, simple diet were added. Easton, "On Longevity," mentions one Numas de Cugna, a native of Bengal, who died in 1566, at the astonishing age of 370 years; he also quotes two respectable Portuguese authors, in support of the fact. However favorable a northern climate may be to longevity, too great a degree of cold is, on the other hand, prejudicial to it. The medium, rather inclining to cold, with some degree of civilization, are best suited to the full development of the physical organs, and also to longevity. In Iceland, and the northern parts of Asia, such as Siberia, men attain, at most, to the age only of sixty or seventy. But besides England and Scotland, Ireland is celebrated for the longevity of its inhabitants; and we doubt not, henceforth, having taken the advice of Father Mathew, and are now banishing the reptiles, strong drinks, from their beautiful green isle, it will be still more celebrated. St. Patrick is said to have banished all natural reptiles from their shores; but Father Mathew is conferring a still greater boon on his country, by banishing artificial ones, in the shape of whisky, etc. May he go on and prosper! As a proof of the longevity of Irishmen, we observe that, in Dunsford, a small place in that country, there were living, at one time, eighty persons above the age of fourscore; and Lord Bacon says there was not a village in the whole island, as he believed, in which there was not one man upward of eighty. In France, instances of longevity are not so abundant; though a man died there, in 1757, at the age of 121. The case is the same in Italy; yet, in the northern provinces of Lombardy, there have been some instances of great age. In Spain, also, there have been instances, though seldom, of men who lived to the age of 110. That healthy and beautiful country, Greece, is still as celebrated as it was formerly, in regard to longevity. Tournefort found, at Athens, an old consul, who was 118 years of age. The island of Naxos is particularly celebrated on this account. Even in Egypt and India, there are instances of long life, particularly among the vegetarian Bramins, anchorites, and hermits, who detest the indolence and intemperance of the other inhabitants of those countries. Ethiopia formerly was much celebrated for the longevity of its inhabitants; but a very different account is given by Bruce, as to its present condition, showing that climate is not the only prerequisite for longevity, as that cannot have been altered much. Some districts of Hungary are distinguished by the great age of the people who reside in them. Germany contains abundance of old people; but it affords few

3*

instances of very long life. Even in Holland, people may become old; though this is not often the case, as few live there to the age of 100 years.

On the whole, then, it will be found to be an incontrovertible fact, that the more a man follows and is obedient to those laws which the all-wise Ruler of the universe has established for his guidance, the longer will he live, other things being equal; and, though this is a general law, it is not so much the effect of climate as the mode of living. In the same districts, therefore, as long as the inhabitants lead a temperate life, they will attain to old age; but as soon as they become highly civilized, and by these means sink into luxury, dissipation, and corruption, which is commonly the case, their health will suffer, and their lives be shortened. In the course of nine years' advocacy of the temperance cause, we have often met with objections to our views of intemperance in eating and drinking being destructive of health and longevity; and we are ready to admit that there are exceptions to the rule; but they are so rare as to be *only* exceptions, and not the rule. Yet, we are certain, had those persons who, by more than usually good constitutions, have lived to seventy or eighty years, adopted a rational mode of living, they would have been honored with ranking with our Jenkinses, Parrs, and Cams; and instead of being distinguished, in their latter days, by palsied limbs, by racking pains, an intellect betokening a state of dotage, and, as Bishop Berkely observes, being set up as the devil's decoys,* to draw in proselytes, they would have sunk into the grave as into a sweet repose, at the close of a long, useful, and happy

* Dr. Cheyne mentions one of these decoys, who had drank from two to four bottles of wine every day, for fifty years, and boasted that he was as hale and hearty as ever. "Pray," remarked a bystander, "where are your boon companions?" "Ah!" he quickly replied, "that's another question: if the truth may be told, I have buried three entire generations of them." And, as Dr. Beddoes observes, "Neither do all who are exposed to its contagion, catch the plague; and yet is the hazard sufficient to induce every man in his sober senses [when is the drunkard in his?] to keep out of the way of infection."

life, and perhaps been enabled, to the very last, to relish the enjoyments of reason. Thus, instead of decoying others into bad ways, they would have been able to communicate to them the lessons of wisdom, which they had been taught by long personal experience and observation. (See Appendix, D.)

The above facts, to which we have called attention, are all derived from unimpeachable and, as regards our object, from disinterested sources; and are of such an unequivocal nature, that we may confidently base our system upon them, as to its influence on health and longevity. If, however, they fail to convince, even the least skeptical, we think we may safely adopt the language of Abraham to the rich man, "neither will they be persuaded, though one rose from the dead."

CHAPTER IV.

DEATH.

It is a common argument among divines in the behalf of religious life, that a contrary behavior has such consequences when we come to die! It is indeed true, but seems an argument of a subordinate kind; the article of death is more frequently of short duration. Is it not a stronger persuasive, that virtue makes us happy daily, than that it smooths the pillow of a death-bed?—SHENSTONE.

MANY of our readers on closing the book, after reading the remarks in the preceding chapter, will perhaps exclaim, "We do not wish to live so long!" Perhaps not. And how many there are who feel in their old age, as did Louis Wholeham, at the age of 118, less resigned to die than he was eighty years before. Even the Christian who has "a good hope through grace," and knows that "if the earthly house of his tabernacle were dissolved, he has a house not made with hands, eternal in the heavens;" even he fees the physician at no small cost, and takes the most nauseous drugs to ward off the "last enemy." One reason for this anxiety probably is, that the evening of the longest day finds most men with their work but imperfectly done, and therefore but ill prepared for their final account. Besides, as we are not isolated beings, we cannot sever the bond which unites us to the whole human family; and therefore we eat not to ourselves—we drink not to ourselves—we live not to ourselves—we die not to ourselves. "Living or dying we are the Lord's," and are bound to take care that we do not, by indulgence or neglect, render that body a mass of disease and infirmity, and useless to him and his church on earth. The lame, the blind and the maimed, among the Jews, were neither received as a sin-offering or a peace-offering. We owe to God, his church, and the world, the longest and the best life we can live, and are under the most solemn obligations not to injure or shorten it. "Do thyself no harm," and "Thou shalt not kill," are among the positive laws of Jehovah, still binding on the conscience of all; and he "will not hold him guiltless" who violates them. They form a part of that great standard by which, in the day of judgment, every man's actions will be tried. Their design is obvious. Like all other divine commands or prohibitions, they state the rights either of God or of his creatures; and demand a regard to those rights on pain of eternal death. One command guards one precious interest, another presents and defends another. The prohibitions before us refer to two of our dearest interests—our HEALTH and our LIFE. They are both the gift of God. Most tenderly has he guarded, most sternly does he threaten, and most dreadfully will he punish every earthly invader who dares lift up his hand against them, or who carelessly injures them.

But still we are dying creatures, and though by proper attention, and the due observance of those laws which pertain to life and health, we may greatly promote both, yet "it is appointed unto man once to die." This is the purpose of God—the decree of Jehovah. While, therefore, we are concerned to live well and long, let us be equally anxious to die well and happy. This is of great importance physically; as no one who had a great fear of dying ever attained to a great age. But it is of infinitely more importance morally; for, though a man dies, he shall "live again," either in happiness or woe.

> "Since then we die but once, and after death
> Our state no alteration knows,
> But when we have resigned our breath,
> The immortal spirit goes
> To endless joys or everlasting woes;
> Wise is the man who labors to secure
> That mighty and important stake,
> And by all methods strives to make
> His passage safe, and his reception sure.

Let the reader remember, that if by temperance, etc., he should secure health and long life, and should nevertheless neglect his soul, it will profit him nothing. All earthly blessings, even health and life, though among the greatest, have only the condition of an annuity for life; and as such, each succeeding year makes a considerable decrease in their value; and at death the whole is at an end forever. But not so with the man who has "fled for refuge" to the world's Redeemer—has found "redemption in his blood, and the forgiveness of sins"—is "justified by faith"—"has peace with God"—"the love of God shed abroad in his heart by the Holy Ghost given unto him." He dies in peace! And can it be otherwise? Having obeyed the organic laws, he dies, not of disease and racking pain, but of old age. Having experienced "repentance toward God, and faith in our Lord Jesus Christ;" and having obtained "grace to help him in time of need," he has "finished his course of joy," and is now about to receive "the crown of life which the Lord has promised to those that love him." His death-bed is, therefore, a glorious place. The heavens are serene—his anchorage is good, having entered within the veil; he knows his future inheritance is secured by the death of Christ—therefore we need not wonder that

> "The chamber, where the good man meets his fate,
> Is privileged beyond the common walk
> Of virtuous life, quite on the verge of heaven."

With him all is calm and serene. Behind him all is sprinkled with atoning blood. Around him all is conquered. Before him all is fraught with good—rich, boundless, and eternal. No wonder, then, that he should die in peace, for he has no guilt to torment him; "being justified by faith" he has peace with God. Death cannot terrify him, for its sting is taken away—nor is there any thing in eternity to create anxiety for the "*judge is his friend.*" Thus

> "You see the man; you see his hold on heaven,
> Through nature's wreck, through vanquished agonies;
> Like the stars struggling in this midnight gloom;
> What gleams of joy! What more than human peace!

Where the frail mortal, the poor abject worm?
No, not in death the mortal to be found.
His conduct is a legacy for all,
Richer than Mammon's for their single hire.
His comforters he comforts; GREAT IN RUIN."

Still there are thousands who could subscribe to all we have said above, as to the comforts of God's people in dying circumstances, who are, nevertheless, "through fear of death, all their lifetime subject to bondage." This in the Christian arises in most cases from a mistaken notion respecting the actual separation of the soul from the body in the article of death. An eminent author has very justly said—"No man certainly ever felt what death is; and as insensibly as we enter into life," supposing there be no guilt on the conscience, "equally insensibly do we leave it. The beginning and the end are here united. My proofs are as follows: First, no man can have any sensation of dying; for to die, means nothing more than to lose the vital power; and it is the vital power by which the soul communicates sensation to the body. In proportion as the vital power decreases, we lose the power of sensation, of consciousness; and we cannot lose life without at the same time, or rather before, losing our vital sensation, which requires the assistance of the tenderest organs.* We are taught also by experience, that all those who ever passed through the first stage of death, as in cases of partial drowning, etc., and were again brought to life, unanimously asserted that they felt nothing of dying, but sunk at once into a state of insensibility." The same author cautions us against being led into error on this subject, "by the convulsive throbs, the rattling in the throat, and the apparent pangs of death,

* Death, of all estimated evils, is the only one whose presence never incommoded any body, and which only causes concern during its absence. —*Arcesilaus.* There is nothing terrible in death but what our lives have made so; hence many a Christian has been able to say, with Dr. Goodwin, "Is this dying? Is this the enemy that dismayed me so long—now appearing so harmless—and even pleasant?"

which are observed in many persons in a dying state. These symptoms are painful to the spectators, and not to the dying, who are not sensible of them. The case is the same as if one, from the dreadful contortions of a person in an epileptic fit, should come to a conclusion respecting his internal feelings. This would be evidently wrong; for, from what affects us so much, he suffers nothing." If, therefore, we have imbibed the spirit of the sweet singer of Israel, and can say of his "Shepherd," "He restoreth my soul; he leadeth me in paths of righteousness for his name's sake;" let us also say, "Yea, though I walk through the valley of the shadow of death, I will fear no evil, for thou art with me thy rod and thy staff they comfort me."

"To die, is landing on some peaceful shore,
Where billows never beat, nor tempests roar;
Ere well we feel the friendly stroke, 'tis o'er."—*Garth.*

PART II.

CHAPTER V.

GENERAL EFFECTS OF DIET OF THE HUMAN SYSTEM.

Providence has gifted man with reason; to this, therefore, is left the choice of his food and drink, and not to instinct, as among the lower animals. It thus becomes his duty to apply his reason to the regulation of his diet; to shun excess in quantity, and what is noxious in quality; to adhere, in short, to the simple and the natural; among which the bounty of his Maker has afforded him an ample selection; and beyond which, if he deviates, sooner or later he will suffer the penalty.

PROUT'S BRIDGEWATER TREATISE.

THE vital principle, which we call life, though modified by peculiar circumstances, is the same in all human beings. It becomes, therefore, of importance that these circumstances should be understood by us, because, as we have seen in the chapter on "Health and Longevity," this principle can only be secured in a healthy state for many years by the regular and harmonious action of all the functions of the system. It is subject to, and a consequence of, a due performance of the organic laws. Proper food, water, air, exercise, and rest, with entire abstinence from drugs, are essential to its continuance. Every circumstance which tends to enfeeble the organic functions, diminishes, in a greater or less degree, the force of the vital functions.

A little attention to the subject of diet will be sufficient to show how much health and longevity depend upon a proper line of conduct in this respect; inasmuch as the whole constitution of our bodies may be changed by it alone: nor is it less important in the cure of disease. Hence, it is truly astonishing that Priessnitz, that man of nature, should be so much influenced by the gross mode of living generally adopted by the Germans.* The manner in which this matter is handled by Mr. Claridge (See Appendix, E.), in his otherwise excellent work, is a great drawback on its merits and usefulness. Yet there is much in Priessnitz's system of diet which is very excellent; such as taking their aliments cold, etc.

The object of food being to supply the system with nutriment, health in a great measure depends on a proper supply† of the best quality. This is also of great importance mentally as well as physically; for as Dr. Cheyne justly observes, "He that would have a clean head must have a clean body." The stomach, which has been denominated by Lord Bacon "the father of the family;" and by J. J. Gurney, Esq., "the kitchen of the house," is the centre of sympathy, and intimately connected with the body and the mind; the most important organ in the preservation, or the restoration of health; is capable of modifying the action of every substance submitted to it; and if either the body or mind be hurt, intelligence of the injury is soon carried to it, and it soon becomes distended and offenced,‡ in proportion to the importance of

* We are informed by those who have visited Graefenburg, that patients are provided with the veal of calves not more than a day or two old. Hares, coarse, dry, or tough, being first boiled, and then baked. Pork, goose, duck and sausages, all baked, help to vary the repast. Add to this, old mutton and cow beef, stewed in vinegar, succeeded by rancid ham, served up with mashed grey peas. They have also cucumbers cured in nothing but salt and water, which the Germans devour with avidity; yet wonders are effected, proving the efficacy of the water treatment.

† The invigorated state, which in two or three years would ensue, on a return to the laws of nature, the appetite would measure the quantity of vegetable food proper to be taken during the day; an advantage which is lost at a well-furnished table, where the flavor of the dishes is too seductive for us to recollect the juice of the meat that has been compressed for our destruction. Return to nature.

‡ The stomach, that great organ, soon,
If overcharged, is out of tune;

the part, and the degree in which it is hurt; this injury is resented either by excess of languor or excitement—doing too little in the first case, and too much in the latter. In the one case constipation, and in the other diarrhœa is increased, in such as are subject thereto; and all chronic complaints are exasperated. The habits of society very much contribute to this state of things. The quantity* of food commonly made use of by those who can get it, its innutritive qualities, and the almost endless variety of dishes, tend very much to injure the functions of the stomach, and to frustrate its important operation. These people think the more plentifully they stuff themselves, the better they must thrive, and the stronger they must grow; forgetting, if they ever knew, that it is not the quantity taken into the stomach, but that which is properly digested and assimilated, which nourishes and strengthens—all besides this weakens.

Food is of two kinds, solid and liquid; and important as the subject is, still no specific, but only general, rules can be laid down for its use. It is very difficult to ascertain the exact quantity, etc., of food proper for every sex, age, constitution, and condition of life; nor is such a nicety at all necessary, ex-

Blown up with wind that sore annoys
The ear, with most unhallow'd noise!
Now all these sorrows and diseases
A man may fly from, if he pleases;
For early rising will restore
His powers to what they were before;
Teach him to dine at nature's call,
And to sup lightly, if at all;
And leave the folly of night dinners
To fools, and dandies, and old sinners.

* It is your superfluous second courses, and ridiculous variety of wines, ices, desserts, etc., which are served up, more to gratify the appetite and pamper the pride of the host, than to promote the health of those who partake thereof; it is these which overcome the stomach and paralyze digestion, and seduce children of larger growth to sacrifice the health and comfort of several years for the baby pleasures of tickling their tongues for a few minutes with champagne, custards, and trifles.

cept in extreme cases, which will never occur to the man of nature. Mankind were never intended to weigh and measure their food; they have a better standard to go to—honest instinct,* which seldom fails to make out a title to be called unerring. Our stomachs are, in general, pretty good judges of what is best for them, if we would allow them to guide us. Thousands have perished for being inattentive to their call, for one who has implicitly obeyed them. Yet nothing is more common than for invalids to inquire of their medical attendant what food is proper for them. What nonsense! Their doctor might with more propriety be required to tell them what was most agreeable to their palates.† "A fool or a physician at forty," is an adage containing more truth than is commonly believed. He who has not by that time learned to observe the causes of self-disorder, shows few signs of wisdom; and he who has carefully noted down‡ the things which create disorder in himself, must possess much knowledge, which a physician at

* The horse or the ox which declines Harrowgate waters, is wiser than man; nature has made the waters nauseous to warn all animals against drinking it; the animal, therefore, which follows instinct, is right; the reasoning animal, man, is wrong.—*Times.*

Prompted by instinct's never-erring power,
Each creature knows its proper aliment.
Directed, bounded by this power within,
Their cravings are well-aimed:
Voluptuous man
Is by superior faculties misled;
Misled from pleasure even in quest of joy.—*Armstrong.*

† A Dutchman who had been a long time in the free use of ardent spirits, was at length persuaded to give them up, and to join a temperance society. A few months after, feeling unwell—a sinking at the stomach—he sent for a doctor, who prescribed for him, an ounce of spirits. Not understanding what an ounce was, he asked a friend, who told him eight drachms make an ounce. Ah! exclaimed the Dutchman, the doctor understands my case exactly; I used to take six drachms (small glasses) in a day, and I always wanted two more.

‡ Locke says, "Were it my business to understand physic, would not the surer way be to consult nature itself in the history of diseases and their cure, than to espouse the principles of the dogmatists or chemists?"

a pop visit ought not to pretend to.* But if we could lay down specific rules, as to the kind and quality, and also the time of taking food, there would be two grand obstacles in the way of accomplishing our object: 1. They are not always under our control. 2. Few have moral courage enough to war against appetite and adopt them, even when they commend themselves to their judgment.

"But alas, these are subjects on which there's no reasoning;
For you'll still eat your goose, duck, or pig,† with its seasoning;
And what is far worse—notwithstanding its huffing,
You'll make for your hare and your veal a good stuffing.
And I fear if a leg of good mutton you boil,
With sauce of vile capers that mutton you'll spoil;
And though, as you think, to preserve good digestion,
A mouthful of cheese is the best thing in question,
In Gath do not tell it, nor in Askalon blab it,
You're strictly forbidden to eat a Welsh rabbit."

* I never yet met with any person of common sense (except in acute illness), whom I did not think much fitter to choose for himself than I was to determine for him.—*Dr. Heberden.*

† Nothing is more common than for people to take (because advised by the doctor) a rasher of broiled or fried bacon for breakfast to cure the heartburn. (See Appendix, F.) The practice is almost too absurd to be reasoned upon. We have induced several to abandon it, with good effect. For though a small portion may not do much harm to persons who have to go to plough, or to thrash in the barn all day, to studious and sedentary persons, who have little exercise and fresh air, it must be injurious. But we are told that working men, who are the most healthy class of the community, eat bacon and pork. We ask how much of it? Not so much per month as some eat in a day; besides the fact, that they often work from twelve to sixteen hours per day in the pure open air, by means of which, and the perspiration, they throw off its noxious particles.

CHAPTER VI.

ON SOLID FOOD.

If a regular and reasonable mode of life be of such importance to the healthy and robust, how much more essential must it be for weakly persons and invalids! We are justified in asserting, that no cure can be effected without a suitable and natural diet.*—DR. WEISS.

ALL solid food is either of animal or vegetable origin; and difference of opinion prevails as to whether of the two, or an admixture of both, be best adapted to the constitution of man. As we do not wish to lead our readers blindfold—because we believe in the force of truth—we will lay before them the substance of what has been said on both sides of the question, in order that they may judge for themselves, as we have.†

In favor of animal food, it has been asserted that it is more allied to our nature, and more easily assimilated to its nourishment; that it is highly favorable to corporeal exertion;‡ that

* The choice and measures of the materials of which our bodies are composed, and what we take daily by pounds, is at least of as much importance as what we take seldom, and only by grains and spoonfuls.—*Dr. Arbuthnot.*

† The author was, in part, a carnivorous animal when he commenced these sheets, but became wholly an herbivorous and frugivorous one before he had finished them. *Magna est veritas!*

‡ Are not the Irish, who live almost exclusively on potatoes and buttermilk, as strong as any race of men in Europe? It is notorious that they are vigorous, even to a proverb; so that if a man remarkable for the large ness of his limbs be exhibited in London, it is ten to one but he comes from the sister kingdom. We find also, in Ulloa's book on South America, that men may be abundantly sustained on vegetables. He tells us that "instances are common," on that continent, "of persons in good health at one hundred and thirty or forty years of age." The habits of the Spaniards are very different from ours. And we are told by travelers, that it is astonishing what a distance a Spanish attendant will accompany, on

we can subsist upon it much longer without becoming hungry; and because it consists of parts which have already been digested by the proper organs of an animal, it only requires solution and mixture, whereas vegetable food must be converted into the substance of an animal nature by the proper action of our own viscera, and therefore requires more labor of the stomach, and other digestive organs.* (See Appendix, G.) For these reasons it is said the dyspeptic, the bilious, and the nervous, whose organs of digestion are weak, find in general animal food the most suitable; that men inhabiting northern regions, where the system is liable to be weakened, and even exhausted, by extreme temperature, and especially by the depressing agency of cold,† a large quantity of animal food is required, as being more stimulating and invigorating. It is also said, that considered anatomically, man is evidently designed to live on animal food, at least in parts.‡ And lastly, it is argued that na-

foot, a traveler's mule or carriage—not less than forty or fifty miles a day—raw onions and bread being his only fare.

* Dr. Cheyne has combated this notion, and asserts that the jelly—the juices or chyle of animal substances—is infinitely more tenacious and gluey (vide "Memoirs of the Academy Royal," for 1729 and 1730), and its last particles more closely united, and separated with greater difficulty, than those of vegetable substances. The flesh of animals, I say, must with far greater difficulty be digested and separated. As a proof of which, is it not said in favor of animal food, that a person can go longer on it than he can on vegetables? Yes! because the former is not so easily or so soon digested, or cleared off the stomach.

† This is, perhaps, the best reason of the whole, if it be applied to cases in an extremely cold climate. (See Appendix, H.) Hence the Russian will consume his three pounds of tallow, and three quarts of train oil per day, which contain about sixty per cent. of carbon—and which is also about the per centage of fat bacon and ham.

‡ This is a most unfortunate argument in favor of animal food, because the reverse is notoriously the fact. Comparative anatomy teaches us that man resembles frugivorous and herbivorous animals in every thing, and carnivorous animals in nothing; he has neither claws wherewith to seize or hold his prey, nor distinct and pointed teeth, to tear the living fibre, as is the case with the lion, tiger, wolf, dog, cat, etc.; the vulture, owl, hawk, etc. It is only by softening and disguising dead flesh by culi-

ture seems to have provided other animals for the use of man, from the astonishing increase of some sorts.*

Against a vegetable diet it has been argued, that it has a constant tendency to sourness; is not so easily assimilated to our nature; distends the stomach by the quantity of air which it contains, and which is extricated or let loose by the warmth of the stomach;† that it does not contain so large a proportion of nutriment,‡ and is not, therefore, so nutritious and invigorating as animal food; and that vegetables of the pulse kind are liable to strong objections as articles of diet by civil-

nary preparations, that it is rendered susceptible of mastication and digestion, and that the sight of its bloody juices and raw horus do not excite intolerable loathing and disgust. The orang-outang perfectly resembles man, both in the order and number of his teeth, and is the most anthropomorphous of the ape tribe, which are strictly frugivorous. This animal, which lives on fruits and vegetables, is so vigorous, that when first taken it requires half a dozen men to hold him. Formerly those who had the care of them in menageries, etc., fed them on flesh, from which they have now ceased, or nearly so, because it rendered them gross and shortened their lives. There is no other species of animals, which live on different food, in which this analogy exists. In many frugivorous animals the canine teeth are more pointed and distinct than those of man. The resemblance also of the human stomach and that of the "Man of the Woods," is greater than that of any other animal. The intestines are also identical with those of herbivorous animals, which presents a large surface for absorption, and have ample and cellulated colons. The cæcum also, though small, is larger than that of carnivorous animals; and even here, the orang-outang retains its accustomed similarity. See more on this subject in *Cuvier*, Lecons d'Anat. Comp. tom. iii. etc. *Rees*, Cyclop., Man.

* So large is the increase of pigeons, that in the space of four years 14,760 may come from a single pair; and in the same time, 1,274,840 from a pair of rabbits. But it should be remembered, that the increase of animals, as also the production of a certain amount of any kind of vegetable food, depends, to a large extent, on the will of man. Hence we sometimes obstruct this increase.

† This is true of cabbage, greens, etc., which are fit, as articles of diet, for cows, pigs, etc. Nevertheless, this distension of the stomach, to some extent, is essential.

‡ From analyses by experienced chemists—such as MM. Percy, Van-

ized man,* as being very indigestible, at least to all but the robust, etc. (See Appendix, I.)

On the other hand, it has been argued in favor of a vegetable diet, and against animal food, that in temperate climates, like ours, an animal diet is more wasting than a vegetable, because it excites, by its stimulating properties, a temporary fever after each meal made of it, by which the springs of life are urged into constant preternatural and weakening exertion; that persons who live chiefly on animal food are subject to determination of blood to the head,† to corpulency, and to various acute and fatal disorders, as the scurvy, malignant ulcers, inflammatory fevers, etc.; and that there appears in this mode

guielin, etc.—it is found that the proportion of nutritious matter, in some of the most common human aliments, is as follows:

Gross Weight. lbs.	Kind of Food.	Net amount of nutritious matter. lbs.
100	Lentiles (dry), ...	94
"	Peas (dry), ...	93
"	Beans (dry), ...	89 to 90
"	Wheat, ...	85
"	Barley, ...	83
"	Rye, ...	80
"	Rice, ...	80
"	Bread, ...	80
"	Flesh (average), ...	35
"	Potatoes, ...	25
"	Beet Root, ...	14
"	Carrots, ...	10
"	Cabbage, ...	7
"	Greens, ...	6
"	Turnips, ...	4

* Not so, then, it seems to the man of nature, who only eats to answer the demands of nature, and not merely to gratify his appetite.

† If adopting a vegetable diet should occasion considerable paleness and shrinking of features for a time, it is no bad sign, and is not essential to the system, as young children who are so brought up have a fine color in the second year, and enjoy perfect health and considerable strength. Nor should such paleness, etc., excite our apprehension, since the vessels being less loaded, it is thus the determination of blood to the head is prevented.

of living a strong tendency to promote the formation of many chronic diseases, as we seldom see those who indulge in this diet, remarkable for health and longevity. Besides, it is said a man could not live entirely upon animal food,* but he could on vegetables; and a vegetable diet, when it consists of articles easily digested—such as bran bread,† pulse, Scotch oatmeal, potatoes, plain puddings, rice, etc.—is highly favorable to longevity.

There are also instances of persons making great exertion with this aliment. Dr. R. Jackson says, "I have wandered a good deal about the world, and never followed any prescribed rules in any thing; my health has been tried in all ways; and by the aid of temperance and hard work, I have worn out two armies, in two wars, and probably could wear out another before my period of old age arrives. *I eat no animal food, drink no wine, or malt liquor, or spirits of any kind;* I wear no flannel, and neither regard wind nor rain, heat nor cold, where business is in the way." This food has also a most beneficial influence on the mental powers, and tends to preserve a delicacy of feeling, a liveliness of imagination, and an acuteness of judgment, seldom enjoyed by those who live chiefly on flesh. Dr. Cullen observes of vegetable diet, that it never over-distends the vessels, or loads the system—"never interrupts the stronger motions of the mind; while the heat, fullness, and weight of animal food, is an enemy to its vigorous efforts." The celebrated Dr. Franklin, partly on the recommendation of Tryon, and partly on the ground of economy, took entirely to a vegetable diet. His frugal meals frequently consisted of only a biscuit, or a slice of bread and bunch of raisins, or a bun with a glass of water. At one time, he and another printer at Philadelphia spent only *eighteen pence per week*, in diet, between them; and he mentions that his progress in study was propor-

* The late Sir E. Barry prevailed upon a man to live eight days on partridges, without vegetables; but he was obliged to desist, from the appearance of strong symptoms of putrefaction.

† Bread made of flour having only the broad bran taken out of it.

tioned to that clearness of ideas, and quickness of conception, which are the fruits of temperance in eating and drinking. It also further appears that animal food is more easily carried to excess; has a continual tendency in it, as has also the human body itself, to putrefaction; fills the blood-vessels, and loads the brain, which causes heaviness and stupor, and lays the foundation of disease; in particular, corpulency, obesity, and putrescent acrimony. Animal food is less adapted to the sedentary than the laborious, and least of all to the studious, whose diet ought to consist of vegetables. Volney, in his "Travels," speaking of the Wallachians, says: "They are in general tall, well built, and of very wholesome complexion. Diseases are very rare among them," and that "their manners, so far as I have been able to judge of them, are simple. Temperate in their repasts, they prefer vegetables to fruits, and fruits to the most delicate meats." Sir W. Temple, speaking of the ancient Bramins, says: "Their temperance was so great that they lived upon rice or herbs, and on nothing that had sensitive life. If they fell ill, they counted it such a mark of *intemperance*, that they would frequently die out of shame and sullenness; but many lived a hundred and fifty, and some, two hundred years.

Rousseau, speaking of the moral effect of aliment, says, it is "clearly evinced in the different tempers of the carnivorous and the frugivorous animals; the former, whose destructive passions, like those of ignorant men, lay waste all within their reach, are constantly tormented with hunger, which returns and rages in proportion to their own devastation. This creates that state of warfare or disquietude, which seeks, as in murderers, the night and veil of the forest; for, should they appear on the plain, their prey escapes, or, seen by each other, their warfare begins. The frugivorous animals wander tranquilly on the plains, and testify their joyful existence, by frisking and basking in the conjugal rays of the sun, or browsing, with convulsive pleasure, on the green herb, evinced by the motion of the tail, or the joyful sparkling of the eye, and the gambols of the herds."

The same effect of aliment is seen among the different species of men; and the peaceful temper of the frugivorous Asiatic is strongly contrasted with the ferocious temper of the carnivorous European.*

Moreover, it is notorious, that the nations which subsist on vegetable diet are of all men the handsomest, the most robust, the least exposed to disease, and violent passions, and attain longevity: such are, in Europe, a great portion of the Swiss.

The negroes, doomed to labor so severely, live entirely on manise, potatoes, and maize.

From the Pythagorean school, Epaminondas, so celebrated

* The Tartars, whom Gibbon callsun feeling, bloodthirsty murderers, and who live almost wholly on animal food, are exceedingly ferocious and cruel; while the Bramin and Hindoo, who live entirely on a vegetable diet, are altogether as gentle and mild; proving that—

"All are not savages—come, ye gentle swain,
Like Brama's healthy sons, on Indus' banks,
Whom the pure streams and garden-fruit sustain,
Ye are the sons of nature! Your mild hands
Are innocent."—*John Dyer.*

Who will assert, as asks a popular writer, that, had the populace of Paris satisfied their hunger at the ever-furnished table of vegetable nature, they would have lent their brutal suffrage to the proscription-list of Robespierre? Could a set of men, whose passions were not perverted by unnatural stimuli, look with coolness on an *auto da fe?* Is it to be believed that a being of gentle feelings, rising from his meal of roots and vegetables, would take delight in sports of blood? Was Nero a man of temperate life? Did Muley Ismael's pulse beat evenly? Though history has decided none of these questions, a child could hardly hesitate to answer in the negative. Surely the bile-suffused cheek of Bonaparte, his wrinkled brow, and yellow eye, the ceaselessness and inquietude of his nervous system, speak no less plainly the character of his ambition than his murders and victories. It is next to impossible, had Bonaparte descended from a race of vegetable-eaters, that he could have had either the inclination or the power to ascend the throne of the Bourbons. It is such a man, with violent passions, blood-shot eyes and swollen veins, occasioned by the stimuli of flesh and alcohol, that alone can fight a woman, make a hell of domestic life, and destroy his fellow-man by wholesale. We commend this subject to the attention of all who are opposed to licensed murder.

for his skill in mechanics, and Milo, of Crotona, for his strength, copying the virtues of their founder, who was allowed to be the first-rate genius of his day, and the father of philosophy among the Greeks.*

The children of the Persians, in the time of Cyrus, and by his orders, were fed with bread, water, and cresses; and Lycurgus introduced a considerable part of the physical and moral regimen of these children into the education of those of of Lacedæmon. Such diet prolongs infancy, and consequently prolongs life. It is also surprising to what a great age the eastern Christians—who retired to the deserts of Egypt and Arabia—lived, on very little food. We are informed, by Cassian, that "the common measure used by them, in twenty-four hours, was about twelve ounces, with mere element to drink."

Haller says, "This food, then, which I have hitherto described, and in which flesh has no share, is salutary, insomuch that it fully nourishes a man, protracts life to an advanced age,† and prevents or cures such disorders as are attributable to the acrimony or grossness of the blood." A physician, in a "Practical Essay," written some hundred years ago, says, "Whoever can resolve, in bad spirits, a bad constitution, and in advanced life, to go into such a regimen, may, I think, fairly be manumitted from drugs."

Mr. Slingsby and Dr. Knight both lived many years on bread, milk, and vegetables, and without intoxicating drinks; they had excellent spirits, and were very vigorous. In fact, hundreds are now pursuing a similar course, with like results. The author of "Vegetable Regimen" gives an account of a

* It is affirmed, by Haller, that Newton, our own great geometrician, wrote his philosophic work, which sheds a lustre on his name and country, on simple bread and water only.

† That animal food and fermented liquors will more readily, certainly, and cruelly create, and exasperate diseases, pains, and sufferings, and sooner cut off life than vegetable food will, there can be no more doubt than any proposition of Euclid, if reason, philosophy, the nature of things or experience have any evidence or force in them.—*Dr. Cheyne.*

number of persons, who have been living upon this diet, ana upon distilled water, for five years past, whose health is so good that "they have no need of medicine, and that, without an exception, their indispositions, where they happen at all, are so trifling as scarcely to deserve the name." He further observes, that "no ill effects have, in any instance, been felt from the adoption of this regimen." To prove how greatly the stomach is fortified, and the digestion improved, by the general increase of health, occasioned by vegetable diet, he says, "that a person thus nourished is enabled to bear what one, whose humors are less pure, may sink under; the children of our family can, each of them, eat twelve or eighteen walnuts, without the most trifling indigestion—an experiment which those who feed their children in the usual manner would consider it adventurous to attempt." (See Appendix, J.) The same author, speaking of the effect of vegetable diet on children, refers to the case of his own, four in number, all under nine years of age, who, he says, had not cost him "one farthing for medicine, or medical attendance, in the course of two years." He also states that several medical men, who had "examined them with a scrutinizing eye, all agreed that they knew nowhere a whole family which equals them in robustness. Their health may be verified by the inspection of any stranger, who shall be disposed to take that trouble." Indeed, it seems to be the opinion of those who have made the experiment in their own circle, and who are therefore the best judges in the case, that the observance of the laws of nature, by children, would greatly improve their health and strength; that their irritability would gradually subside; they would become more robust and beautiful, their carriage be more erect, their step more firm; and that the danger of parents being deprived of them, at an early period, would be much diminished; while, by their light repasts, their hilarity would be greatly augmented, and their intellects cleared, in a degree which would astonishingly illustrate the delightful effect of this regimen.

But we shall be told, by the very people who will blame us

for the reference, that we should go to a higher authority than erring mortals, and submit our theory to the test of Scripture. We will do so, not because we place the weight of our argument there, but because some will seek to condemn our practice from that source. Our forte is in the human, physiological, and moral view of the subject. Our opponents tell us we do wrong in rejecting "the good creatures of God," though they refuse frog soup, etc., etc., which are regarded with so much attachment by other nations; and that in Gen. iii. 9, God gave to Noah and his sons "every living thing that moveth," to be meat for them, "even as the green herb." True, and though nothing is more plain, from nature and its eternal laws, and from justice and equity, than that, in the original intention, one woman was designed for one man, yet, for "the hardness of their hearts," God permitted plurality of women to the Jews; nevertheless, our Lord has declared that "from the beginning* it was not so." This same people, though they had not only God's general and imperceptible providence, as we have now, for their government and direction, but also his miraculous, sensible, and visible presence, to instruct and guide them, yet they applied to Samuel the prophet, saying, "Give us a king to judge us, like all the nations. But the thing displeased Samuel," because he saw that they were rejecting the Lord that he "should not reign over them." The Lord said unto Samuel, "Hearken unto the voice of the people, in all that they say unto thee." Was this sanction? No! God only

* Then God said (Gen. i. 29), Behold I have given you every herb bearing seed, which is upon the face of the whole earth, and every green tree, in which is the fruit of the tree yielding seed, to you it shall be given for meat. It seems from this, says an eminent philosopher, that man was originally intended to live upon vegetables only; and as no change was made in the structure of men's bodies after the flood, it is not probable that any change was made in the article of food. It may also be inferred from this passage, that no creature whatever was originally designed to prey on others; for nothing is here said to be given to any beast of the earth besides green herbs.—*Dr. Priestley.* Though God gave man dominion over all his creatures, he confined him to the green herb for food.

permitted it, that, as good Matthew Henry says, "They might be beaten with their own rod—to prevent something worse," and that it might "serve his own wise purposes, even by their foolish counsels."* To show that the Lord did not approve of their demand, we refer to the above passage, and also to Hosea, xiii. 11; where God says, "I gave them a king in mine anger, and took him away in my wrath." Lastly, we refer to the facts mentioned in Num. ii.; Ps. lxxviii. 30, 31; cvi. 14, 15, where we are informed that they grew weary of their vegetable diet, the manna, the angel's food, of which they spake so disrespectfully, and with which Providence had so graciously fed them; "They soon forgot his works; they waited not for his counsel; but lusted exceedingly in the wilderness, and tempted God in the desert. And he gave them their request; but sent leanness into their souls. But while their meat was in their mouths, the wrath of God came upon them, and slew the fattest of them, and smote down the chosen men of Israel."

Observe how cautiously, and with what amounts to almost a prohibition, the Jewish law directs this permit of animal food, viz., absolutely and positively not to eat the blood of the animal† (in which its most deleterious qualities chiefly consist, and

* Cheyne supposes that animal food and strong liquors were permitted to man to shorten life, in order to prevent the excessive growth of wickedness. Whatever may be thought of this idea, certain it is, man's life became gradually shortened with the introduction of animal food; and of the consumption of which we have no account till after the deluge, a period of 2000 years.

† How those who profess to regard the Bible as the rule of their doctrine and practice, can eat blood, we cannot conceive. Is not the prohibition as binding now as ever it was? The original reason holds as good now, "the blood is the life," and hence it has been sacred, as the great instrument of expiation, and because it was typical of that blood by which we enter into the holiest. It is certain it was not eaten before the deluge, because animal food was not in use. After the deluge it was one of the seven Nohic precepts. It was prohibited at the giving of the law which was renewed under the gospel, in Acts xv. 20, 29. And the command is still scrupulously obeyed by the Oriental Christians, and

because blood globules resist digestion). Now this, in reality and by insinuation, is to say, that since, for the hardness of your hearts, and your unconquerable lusting, you cannot be brought to abstain altogether from animal food, yet because "the blood is the life thereof," and has morbific qualities, you are to drain it as much as possible of all its moisture, and to eat it plain. By this method, animal food will be less pernicious, and will approach very near to vegetables. There is no understanding this permission in any other way, nor is it otherwise to be reconciled to common sense, however both Jews and Christians have at present dwindled and diluted its true import.—*Cheyne.* In reference to the distinction made by Jehovah between the clean and unclean under the law, Dr. A. Clarke says, "While God keeps the eternal interests of man steadily in view, he does not forget his earthly comforts; he is at once solicitous both for the health of his body and his soul. He has not forbidden certain aliments because he is a sovereign, but because he knew they would be injurious to the health and morals of the people. The close connection that subsists between the body and the soul we cannot fully comprehend; and as little can we comprehend the influence which they have on each other. Many moral alterations take place in the mind in consequence of the influence of the bodily organs; and these latter are greatly influenced by the kind of aliment which the body receives. In all this God shows himself the tender Father of a numerous family, pointing out to his inexperienced, froward, and ignorant children those kinds of aliments which he knows

by the whole Greek Church; and why? because the reasons still subsist. If the eaters of blood knew that it affords a very crude, almost indigestible, and unwholesome aliment, they certainly would not, on these physical reasons, leaving moral considerations out of the question, be so much attached to the consumption of that from which they could expect no wholesome nutriment, and which, to render it even pleasing to the palate, requires all the skill of the cook. See much on the subject in an excellent work by Dr. Delaney, entitled "Revelation Examined with Candor," a work of uncommon merit, and too little known, in three small volumes.

will be injurious to their health and domestic happiness, and prohibiting them on pain of his highest displeasure. On the same ground he forbade all fish that have not both fins and scales, such as the conger, eel, etc., which abound in gross juices and fat, which very few stomachs can digest. Who, for instance, that lives solely on swine's flesh* has pure blood and healthy juices? And is it not evident, in many cases, that the man partakes considerably of the nature of the brute on which he exclusively feeds? I could pursue this subject much further, and bring many proofs founded on indisputable facts, but I forbear, for he who might stand most in need of caution, would be the first to take offence."

We have a most pleasing instance of firmness in adhering to their vegetable regimen, in Daniel and his captive companions (Dan. chap. i.). They were put under the care of the master of the eunuchs, and they were "appointed a daily provision of the king's meat, and of the wine which he drank." But they were such rigid teetotalers and vegetarians, that they proposed in their hearts that "they would not defile themselves with the king's meat and wine." Daniel requested, therefore, that they might be allowed to carry out their plan, which appeared so Utopian that the prince of the eunuchs objected, lest, if they were not found looking as well as their

* Dr. A. Clarke is known to have entertained strong prejudices against swine's flesh and tobacco, and is reported to have said on one occasion, "If I were to offer a sacrifice to the devil, it should be a roasted pig, stuffed with tobacco;" and on another occasion, being called upon to ask a blessing at dinner, on which occasion there was a roaster smoking before him, he very solemnly said, "O Lord, if thou canst bless under the Gospel what thou didst curse under the law, bless the pig!" An instance of the savage cannibalism of these animals came under the author's notice not long since. A sow had actually seized a young child, which was playing at the door, and was making off with it, had not the screams of the child brought its mother to its assistance. Pigs are certainly most filthy, ferocious, foul-feeding animals; they are the most subject to cutaneous diseases and putrefaction of any creature, insomuch, that in the time of a plague, they are universally destroyed by all wise nations, as we do mad dogs.

companions,* it might occasion him the loss of his head. This was a serious matter! Daniel, however, had none of those fears; he knew the merits of the plan proposed, and therefore says, "Prove us for ten days," allowing us nothing but "pulse to eat (that is, peas, lentiles, etc.), and water to drink." The trial was accordingly made, and proved most triumphant; for, at the end of ten days, they were not only no worse, but very much better, "fairer and fatter in flesh,"† of a more beautiful look, and better complexion than "all those which did eat the portion of the king's meat." In addition to which, their intellects were kept clear and vigorous; so that, "in all matters of wisdom and understanding that the king inquired of them, he found them ten times better than all the magicians and astrol-

* People will not believe the benefit of a vegetable diet, nor how much it contributes to the health of the body, unless they try it.

† Dr. Higgingbottom says, A person fat in flesh (that is, in muscle) is beautiful in countenance; so Daniel was; every lineament of the features may be seen in perfection; the muscles give expression to the countenance. Not so with the gross, whose lineaments, which ought to give beauty to the countenance, are filled up, or effused with fat, and form a large, round face, nearly destitute of expression. Fat persons, if not diseased, are candidates for it. Most persons may get fat, if they would only adopt the course of those of whom Prior speaks: They eat, and drink, and sleep—what then? why, sleep, and drink, and eat again. Some will tell us they should get fat, live how they would, which we question. The plan of Abernethy, to live on sixpence a day, and earn it, or that of Dr. Radcliffe, Keep your eyes open, and your mouth shut (that is, sleep less and eat less), would soon prove the contrary. For, as Dr. Arbuthnot says, You may see an army of forty thousand soldiers, without a fat man; and I dare affirm that, by plenty of rest, twenty out of forty shall grow fat. The portly appearance of landlords of inns, butchers, and butlers, is obviously referable to their high living and moderate exercise. But it is rather remarkable that the legs of these men are seldom fat. They have—

Enlarged body, diminished leg.—*Shakspeare.*

It is the size of the calves of the legs which indicate strength, they being formed of muscle, or red flesh. R. Holker, while he was a drunken soldier, used to pad his stockings to make calves to his legs; but when he became a teetotaler, he got new calves. So have many others.

ogers that were in all his realm." Again, when God was about to prepare his servant Elijah, the greatest and best man of his age, for a forty days' journey through the wilderness, to Horeb, he did not furnish him with animal food, but sent an angel to give him "a cake of bread and a cruse of water;" upon which Jay says, "Nature is content with little, and grace with less. How many disorders arise from excess! A voracious appetite is a judgment; a delicate one an infirmity; a dainty one is a disgrace. Ministers, above all men, should not be given to appetite, or be fond of dainty meat; and those who entertain them should not insult them by the nature and the degree of their preparations." John the Baptist, also, who was spoken of as coming in "the spirit and power of Elias, had his raiment of camel's hair, and a leathern girdle about his loins; and his meal was locusts and wild honey." The locust was the fruit of the locust-tree. Thus we see that He who could as easily have fed John with flesh as with vegetables, frowns not upon the humble fare, but makes it sustain his favorite, and his Son's forerunner. And yet there are hundreds of his servants, now on earth, who speak of vegetable food, and those who choose to live on it, as unworthy of their notice—the latter, in fact, as rejecting the "good creatures of God." But, certain it is, they cannot charge us with cruelty to animals. We say, "Live and let live," which they cannot say; for, according to their notions, if the animal lives, man cannot. Hence, blood must be shed, and the law of God be broken, for their support, in spite of the horrors with which it naturally inspires us. That is not all the evil: life, which has been so greatly curtailed by the use of animal food, is still further abridged by the violence which prevails among the human race, chiefly as the effect which this aliment has upon the passions of man. Man who, in the early ages of the world, and while he was content to live upon vegetable diet, was seen to spare the lives of animals, has accustomed himself no longer to spare even the lives of his fellow-men. If the Almighty intended man should be an animal of prey, how is it that he has implanted within him an instinctive abhorrence of animal torture, and to the shedding of blood? Should not this be man's guide? Some seek to evade the force of this principle, by saying, Animals eat one another, and why may we not eat them? What! if a wolf worries a lamb, does that justify us in doing the same? But, it is still objected, Nature has furnished us with dog-teeth—for what purpose? Surely you are not justified in doing all you have the means of doing! But what is to become of the cattle? We should be eaten up if we were not to destroy them. We say, breed less, and you need not fear the consequence. There is land sufficient for a large increase of men and animals. "England alone, which now contains only about fifteen millions of inhabitants, is capable of producing, by spade husbandry, a sufficiency of nutritive vegetables for the support of one hundred and twenty millions of human beings; but if every one must consume a pound of flesh a day, there is scarcely enough land for the existing population."—*Vegetable Cookery.* If tigers,* wolves, and vultures praise flesh-eating, are we to admit that they speak the truth? Ask a child, even one who has been used to animal food, and is rather fond of it, whether she will go with you into the gar-

* A party of gentlemen from Bombay, one day, visiting the stupendous temple of Elephanta, discovered a tiger's whelp in one of the obscure recesses of the edifice. Desirous of kidnapping the cub, without encountering the fury of its dam, they took it up hastily and retreated. Being left entirely at liberty, and extremely well fed, the tiger grew rapidly, and appeared tame and fondling as a dog, and in every respect entirely domesticated. At length, when having obtained a vast size, and, notwithstanding its apparent gentleness, it began to inspire terror by its tremendous power of doing mischief, it fell in with a piece of raw meat, dripping in the blood. It is to be observed that, up to that moment, it had been studiously kept from raw animal food. The instant, however, it had dipped its tongue in blood, something like madness seemed to have seized the animal; a destructive principle, hitherto dormant, was awakened. It darted furiously, and with glaring eyes, upon its prey; tore it with fury to pieces; and growling and roaring, in the most fearful manner, rushed off toward the dingle.—*Borough Road School-Lesson Book.*

den, to gather some cherries, or to the slaughter-house, to see the ox killed; or, as Dr. Alcott says, "conceive of slaughter and flesh-eating in Eden!"

But we shall be told, "The Saviour eat fish! and his disciples were fishermen!" Granted. And although, as we said before, we do not need references to the Scripture to defend our practice in abstaining from dead flesh; yet we beg to remind those who go to that resource for their defence, that it is possible to be misled by sounds, and from prejudice and custom to form views not exactly in accordance with "the mind of the spirit;" and these views constituting errors in judgment, may lead to errors in practice, which may have a very prejudicial effect on ourselves and on others. We are all too apt to take things for granted, which are not quite self-evident, especially if they suit our inclinations—as in the case of the lovers of strong drink; the slaveholder; and, shall we add, flesh-eaters? We often associate certain ideas with certain forms of speech, which, perhaps, could not be logically borne out. Are you sure this is not the case here? The word fish does not always apply exclusively to an animal, nor does the word fisherman include only one kind of fishers. For we know, in reference to fish, that the Israelites said (Num. xi. 5), "We remember the fish which we did eat freely in Egypt; the cucumbers and the melons, and the onions and the garlick." Herodotus tells us that fish was in common use in his time among the Egyptians; that it was sometimes used fresh and sometimes roasted. Sometimes they dried it in the sun, then beat it small in a mortar, and afterward sifted it through a piece of fine cloth; and thus formed it into cakes, as bread. This is the very way in which the Egyptians now prepare the lotus plant. See "Beauties of Nature and Art Displayed," vol. xii. page 141. Pococke also says, "that when he was in Upper Egypt, they told him that here was a large fish called lotus, which probably is the lotus that was so highly esteemed by the Egyptians." Pinkerton's Col. Parkhurst, in his "Greek Lexicon," says, "It seems not very natural to understand the

Greek word, *opsarion* (John xxi. 9) as signifying fish. It signifies some other kind of provision, of the delicious sort, that may be eaten with bread. Indeed, fish and honey (Luke xxiv. 42) do not seem to be very suitable to be eaten together." In addition to this evidence, Calmet says, "James and John were fishermen with Zebedee their father," and yet "they never ate either fish or flesh." Josephus says no animal fish will live in the Dead Sea, and yet the prophet Ezekiel speaks of an abundance of fishers who should live on its borders. We should recollect also, that when the net brake, while the disciples were fishing, the fish did not escape, which we think they would have done had they been animals. "But it was a miracle! Therefore the fish were kept from getting away." Would it not have been more to the purpose to have preserved the net from breaking? See "Vegetable Cookery." We have before referred to what has been called the "anatomical argument," and believe no intelligent naturalist, or comparative anatomist, will for one moment place himself in competition with Professor Lawrence and Baron Cuvier, and try to prove man a flesh-eater from his structure. We have also spoken of the physiological influence of animal food, and are perfectly satisfied of what Dr. Alcott has said as to the advantage which vegetable-eaters have over others, as to the superior appetite which they enjoy. To be sure he is not always hungry. Indeed, what some people call hunger—a morbid sensation of gnawing—is unknown to him. But there is scarcely a moment of his life, at least when he is awake, in which he could not enjoy the pleasure of eating, even the coarsest viands, with a high relish, provided, however, he knew it was proper for him to eat. Nor is his appetite fickle, demanding this or that particular article, and disconcerted if it cannot be obtained. It is satisfied with any thing which the judgment directs; and though gratified in a high degree by dainties, when nothing better and more wholesome can be obtained, he never craves for them. The vegetable-eater has a more quiet, happy, and perfect digestion, and his food produces better solids and fluids than that of the flesh-eater; it also gives greater solidity and strength to the frame. We have already given cases in confirmation of this statement, and are satisfied if a fair comparison were instituted, the result would be to confirm our views. We say a fair comparison—that is, compare English with English, etc., etc. The vegetable-eater, if temperate in the use of his vegetables (for many greatly err here, supposing they must take large quantities, as they falsely suppose this food less nutritious, which is not the fact, as shown in the table), and if in other respects he conform to the organic laws, will endure, better than the flesh-eater, the extremes of heat and cold, which is allowed to be a sure sign of a good state of health.

Another branch of our subject has been termed the medical; and those who have written on it have asserted, that if health is the best preventive and security against disease, and if a well-selected and properly administered vegetable diet is best calculated to promote and preserve perfect health, then this part of our subject is disposed of at once, and the superiority of the diet we commend is established beyond the possibility of a doubt. Yet, for the sake of some who may doubt our premises, we refer to a few facts. It is now generally known that Howard, the philanthropist, was a vegetable-eater for about forty years, and yet how free from disease, amidst all the contagion with which he was constantly surrounded! The Rev. Josiah Brewer, who is either an abstainer, or rigidly temperate, now a missionary in Smyrna, has been much exposed to disease, and, like Mr. Howard, to the plague itself, and yet we are not aware that he has ever suffered a single day's sickness as the consequence of his exposure. The Rev. Mr. Crocker went out to a sickly part of Africa some years since, and has remained at his station, thus far, in perfect health, while many of his friends have sickened or died. He is a vegetarian. Gen. T. Sheldon, of the United States, also a vegetarian, has spent several years in the most sickly parts of the Southern States, with an entire immunity from disease; and he gives it as his opinion, that it is no matter where we are, so that our dietetic and other habits are correct. Is not this thought worthy of the attention of our missionary committees, and also of our missionaries? Let them try it. Hear also the star, the idol of the British army, Sir R. Sale, who, when sending his dispatches from Jellalabad to the commander-in-chief, says, "I will not mention as a privation, the European troops having been without spirits, because I believe that to be a circumstance tending to keep them in the highest health, and in the most admirable state of discipline; crime has been almost unknown; and a murmur is never heard, although they are deprived of their usual quantity of animal food."

Those who have viewed this matter politically, tell us that the produce of an acre of land in wheat, corn, potatoes, fruit, etc., will sustain animal life sixteen times as long as when the produce of the same acre is converted into flesh by feeding and fattening animals it. But if we admit this estimate is too high, and if the difference is only eight to one, the result may perhaps surprise us; and if we have not done it before, may lead us to reflection. The people of the United States are believed to eat, upon the average, an amount of animal food equal at least to one whole meal a day, and those of Great Britain one in two days. Taking this estimate to be correct, we, by substituting a vegetable for animal food, might sustain forty-nine instead of twenty-one millions of inhabitants, and they fifty instead of fifteen; and this, too, in their present comfort, and without clearing any more land. Here, then, we are consuming that unnecessarily (if animal food is unnecessary) which would sustain sixty-three millions of human beings in life, health, and happiness.

Many people think we ought not to take into consideration the economical bearings of the subject, on the ground of its being mean or parsimonious. But conscious as we are of higher objects, in consulting economy, than the saving of money, that it may be expended on things of more value than the mere indulgence or gratification of the appetites or the passions, in a world where there are drunkards to reclaim, minds to educate, and souls to save, we have ventured to call attention to this subject. We have all heard of "a good garden half supporting a family;" and if a garden of a given size will half support a family, one twice as large would support it wholly. Ten bushels of corn, properly cooked, will support an adult individual a year. Four times this amount is a good allowance for a family of five persons. But how small a spot of good soil is required for raising forty bushels of corn! But as it is perhaps desirable to vary the food, let the cultivator, if he please, raise only twenty bushels of corn, and plant the rest of the ground with peas, potatoes, etc., and he will have abundance, which it would require more than ordinary gluttony to consume.

Notwithstanding we may be told that arguments drawn from experience are fallacious, we must refer to this bearing of the subject, because we differ from our objector—we think it is a proper test. It is a notorious fact that one half of the 900,000,000 of human beings which inhabit our globe live on vegetables, either from necessity or choice; or if they get meat at all, it is so rarely that it can hardly have any effect on their structure or character. In addition to nations and individuals before referred to, we name the Japanese of the interior, who, according to some of the British geographers, live principally upon rice and fruits; and yet they are the finest men in all Asia. The New Hollanders, who eat flesh freely, are not only mere savages, but they are among the most meagre and wretched of the human race. Nearly the same remarks will apply to the Chinese, and with little modification to Hindostan. In short, the hundreds of millions of Southern Asia, are, for the most part, vegetable-eaters; and a large proportion of them live chiefly on rice, though by no means the most favorable vegetable for exclusive use. What countries like these have maintained their ancient, moral, intellectual, and political landmarks? Granted they have made but little improvement from century to century; it is something not to have deteriorated. Let us proceed with our general view of the world, ancient and modern.

The old world were all vegetarians, and the Jews of Palestine nearly so; for though flesh of various kinds was admissible by their law, except at their feasts, and on special occasions, they ate chiefly bread, milk, honey, and fruits.

"The ancient Greeks," says Porphyry, "lived entirely on the fruits of the earth." "The ancient Syrians abstained from every species of animal food." By the laws of Triptolemus, the Athenians were strictly commanded to abstain from all living creatures. Even so late as the days of Draco, the Attic oblations consisted only of the fruits of the earth.

"The Greek historians, when describing the primitive ages of the world, relate that the first race of men regaled themselves on every mild and wholesome herb they could discover, and on such fruits as the trees spontaneously produced; that the food of the primeval generations was different, according to the respective productions of various countries; the ancient Arcadians lived on acorns; the Argives, on pears; the Athenians, on figs. We behold Fabricius, concerning whom the king of Epirus declared, that it was easier to turn the sun from its course, than this venerable patriot from his principles, after having been honored with several triumphs, 'eating,' says Seneca, 'in a corner of his cottage, the pulse he had himself raised and gathered in his garden.' The Romans were so fully persuaded of the superior effects of vegetable diet, that besides the private examples of many of their great men, they publicly countenanced this mode of diet in their laws concerning food; among which were the *Lex Fransua* and the *Lex Licinia*, which, allowing but very little flesh, permitted promiscuously and without limitation all manner of things gathered from the earth, from shrubs, and from trees. Plutarch says, 'It is best to accustom ourselves to eat no flesh at all, for the earth affords plenty enough of things, not only fit for nourishment, but for enjoyment and delight.' And again, 'You ask me for what reason Pythagoras abstained from eating the flesh of brutes? For my part, I am astonished to think, on the contrary, what appetite first induced man to taste of a dead carcass; or what motive could suggest the notion of nourishing himself with flesh of animals which he saw the moment before bleating, bellowing, walking, and looking about them. How could he bear to see an impotent and defenceless creature slaughtered, skinned, and cut up for food? How could he endure the sight of the convulsed limbs and muscles? How bear the smell arising from the dissection? Whence happened it that he was not disgusted and struck with horror when he came to handle the bleeding flesh, and clear away the clotted blood and humors from the wounds? We should therefore rather wonder at the conduct of those who first indulged themselves in this horrible repast, than at such as have humanely abstained from it.'" See this subject treated at large, in an excellent work, "Vegetable Diet Defended," by Dr. W. A. Alcott, which will amply repay for a careful reading. Did our limits permit, we could furnish a list of names, and an array of facts, which would astonish those who have never considered the subject; but we should exceed our bounds, and tire our readers, long before we had exhausted our resources. To those, however, who feel a deep interest in the matter, and have time or patience thoroughly to investigate the subject, we recommend the perusal, among physiologists, of Dr. Graham's "Lectures on the Science of Human Life;" Dr. Combe's "Principles of Physiology Applied to Health;" Hitchcock's "Lectures on Diet," etc.; Combe "On the Constitution of Man." Among physicians, Dr. Alcott, of America; Dr. Cheyne; Sir J. Sinclair; Dr. Taylor; Dr. Abernethy; the celebrated Hufeland, of Germany; Dr. Cullen; Dr. Cranstorne; Dr. Lambe; Dr. Whitlaw, who says, "that all philosophers have given their testimony in favor of a vegetable diet, from Pythagoras to Franklin." We have also quoted from some of the most eminent philosophers and philanthropists, and might have added thereto, from Pythagoras, Plato, Plautus, Plutarch, Porphyry, Lord Bacon, Sir W. Temple,

Cyrus the Great, Lord Kairns, Professor Dick, Sir E. Home, Pope, Sir I. Newton, Sir R. Phillips, Howard, Shelley, Newton, Linnæus, Baron Cuvier, etc.; but their works are before the public, and invite attention.

We are greatly indebted to Dr. Alcott for his "Vegetable Diet Defended," and think his "seven-fold cord" will not "easily be broken;" it is too late in the day of human improvement to meet them with no argument but ignorance, and with no other weapon but ridicule. After all, we think with him, that the moral bearing of the subject is by far the most important. And though the physiological may be deemed the most important by some, yet what great end would be accomplished, even could we bring mankind back to nature's simplicity, if it were only to make them better and more perfect animals; still it would be a point gained; "but after all, we would reform his dietetic habits, principally, to make him better morally; to make him better in the discharge of his varied duties to his fellow-beings and to God. We would elevate him, that he may become as truly godlike or godly as he now too often is, by his unnatural habits, 'earthly, sensual, and devilish.' We would have him a rational being, fitted to fill the space which he appears to have been originally designed to fill—the gap in the great chain of being between the higher quadrupeds and angelic beings—restored to his true dignity—a child of God, and an heir of a glorious immortality."

Having thus fully stated the reasons which have induced us to abandon animal food, and why we wish others to adopt the same course, we leave it, satisfied that if we err, we err on the safe side—we err in company with some of the greatest men that have ever existed in this or any other country—with men with whom it is an honor to be associated. Ours is certainly the oldest—best authorized—most innocent—and most in accordance with humanity, health, and longevity.

CHAPTER VII.

ON LIQUID FOOD.

A mode of life conformable with nature will admit of no other beverage than pure cold water, ordained by her as the common drink for all mankind. To the present day, this law of nature is renounced by the folly, ignorance, aversion, prejudice, and superstition of man. Whenever the voice of nature makes itself heard, it is soon silenced by our sensuality, inclinations, and passions. Many, again, are deficient in sound judgment, or the necessary strength of mind to lay down a prejudice occasionally supported by medical men. There are, moreover, a number of persons, enemies to water from the most improper motives. But all these circumstances are insufficient to conceal the inestimable properties of cold water from quiet and deliberate reason. By the force of conviction, in fact, to which prejudice must yield, correct ideas of the activity of cold water have already gained ground; and we need now no longer doubt their ultimate triumph.—Weiss.

Next to air, liquid food is essential for the support of life; without it no person can exist for any space of time, though instances are not wanting of individuals who have lived long without solid food. We have known several persons living from twenty to thirty days on nothing but cold water. And when we consider how greatly the fluids exceed the solids in the composition of the human body, it has often astonished us that no more attention has been paid to it. It is calculated, by Mead, Keil, Prout, M. le Can, Berzelius, Martin, etc., that there exists, in a healthy condition of the human body, above eighty parts in every one hundred of water—in the chyme more than ninety; in the human blood about seven hundred and eighty parts in every one thousand; in the bile more than nine hundred parts in every one thousand; in the urine above nine hundred and thirty parts in every one thousand; and in the muscle, or the flesh of the animal, more than seventy-seven parts in every one hundred. It must, therefore, be clear, that whether we consider water as an hydroprophylactic (a preventive), or as an hydrotherapeutic (a curative), very much depends upon a free use of it as a drink. If the human frame be, properly speaking, an hydraulic machine (as Mead says it is), contrived with the most exquisite art, in which there are numberless tubes, properly adjusted and disposed, for conveying the fluids to its various parts, it is evident that liquid food is necessary to replace fluids which the body is constantly losing, by perspiration and other means. The time of taking, and also the quantity needed, are indicated by thirst, when the body is in health. Water should be taken, also, at every meal, for the purpose of assisting digestion. (See Appendix, K.) Hence, those who drink little complain of indigestion. It is necessary as a vehicle to convey our solid food from the stomach into all the different parts of the body, in a liquid state; to keep the blood in a sufficient state of fluidity to be circulated throughout the smaller vessels; to wash and carry off the saline particles which are constantly accumulating in the body; to clear away the impurities of the blood; to promote the necessary secretions, such as bile, etc.; and to keep the body in a due state of temperature. The liquids in common use are, chiefly, water and milk (which are nature's beverages), tea, coffee, intoxicating drinks, etc. (which are compounded by art). We shall proceed to make a few observations on each of them, observing, in the outset, that art cannot improve upon the production of infinite goodness and wisdom. In support of this, a host of first-rate medical and other authorities might be quoted. We shall give a few, as a sample. Milton says—

> "O madness! to think the use of strongest wines,
> And strongest drink, our chief support of health,
> When God, with these forbidden, made choice to war,
> His mighty champion, strong above compare,
> Whose drink was only from the limpid brook."

No creature besides man seeks artificial liquids, either as a beverage or as a medicine. The brute creation, when thirsty, repair to the brook to quench their thirst, and, when wounded, to assuage their pain. This is the beverage on which the ox fattens, and on which the horse and the elephant grow strong.

Man only despises it, though he has seen his predecessors pay the penalty, in diseased bodies, tortured minds, and early death. These, however, are only modern and partial evils; for history informs us that, in the remotest ages of antiquity, water served as the exclusive beverage of man, and as the sole purifier of his skin, etc. It was the chief remedy which the intuitive instinct of man suggested to him, in all prevalent diseases; and as long as he was acquainted with no other remedy for those purposes, and his life was in accordance with nature, he remained healthy and strong, and attained to longevity. With the progress of time, artificial, mostly warm, beverages and baths, and stimulating food, mostly flattering to the palate, assumed the place of cold water and vegetable food; and the consequences of this luxurious mode of life soon made their appearance. Debility and diseases, of all kinds, now superseded the sense of health, strength, and comfort, which was experienced before. The irritability of the nervous system was augmented; disturbances of the digestive organs, of all the functions of the mind, and of the whole animal economy, were created. Medical men had recourse to stimulating and poisonous drugs, etc., for the purpose of removing those evils, and repairing the shattered systems of their fellow-men. This was only a further encroachment upon nature, and, consequently, proved inadequate to the purpose. Age succeeded to age, and school to school. Many new systems of treating disease, etc., rose, flourished, and fell, because none answered the necessities of the people. Error made way for error, in the practice of drugging, as man departed from the laws of nature; and thus the multitude lay neglected; and, with few exceptions, their progress to the grave was even facilitated by the very means which were used, professedly, to heal and cure them. Happily, there have been, in all ages, a few thinking, independent men, who have dared to think and act for themselves, and who have sought to recall the use of cold water as a beverage, and also as a medicine, from the disuse into which it had fallen, and to lead mankind back to original and natural modes of life. Many of these having left their record behind them, we beg to refer the reader to a few of them, which bear more particularly upon water as a beverage, and as a preventive of disease.

Pindar says, "The best thing is water, and the next gold." Pythagoras strongly recommended the use of cold water to his disciples, to fortify both their body and mind. The Macedonians considered warm water as enervating; their women, after accouchment, were washed in cold water. Virgil called the ancient inhabitants of Italy a race of men hard and austere, who immersed their newly born children in the rivers, and accustomed them to cold water. Charlemagne, aware of the salubrity of cold bathing, encouraged its use throughout his empire, and introduced swimming as an amusement at his court. Dr. Floyer published a work on this subject, 1702; from which period to 1722, it went through six editions in London. Dr. Hancock, in 1772, published an anti-fever treatise, on the use of cold water, which went through seven editions in one year. But the merit of settling the use of cold water on a just principle, belongs to our own countryman, Currie, whose work, published in 1797, upon the efficacy of water, may be considered the scientific base of hydropathy. Tissot, in his "Advice to the People," published in Paris, 1797, shows the importance of cold water. Under the head of "Facts and Figures," chap. iii., reference was made to the Greeks, Romans, Circassians, New Zealanders, American Indians, Bramins, the natives of Scotland, and of Sierre Leone, etc., as remarkable for their health and longevity, chiefly as the result of their free use of water. To these might have been added the Turks, who as Slade remarks in his excellent work, "Records of the East," that notwithstanding their ignorance of medical skill, added to the extreme irregularity of their living, both as it regards diet and exercise, yet they enjoy particularly good health, and he says this anomaly is owing to two causes: first, the religious necessity of washing their arms feet, and necks, from three to five times a day, always with cold water; secondly, by their constant use of the vapor bath; gout, rheumatism, headache, and consumption are unknown in Turkey. In England, nature is known only by name, and till the eyes of many were opened by the diffusion of temperance truth, none but those who were reduced to the last stage of poverty, ever thought of satisfying their thirst with water. Still, even now, there are very few who have carried their principles out in all their legitimate bearings. And perhaps the greatest hindrances in the way of its more extensive use as a beverage, is, it costs us nothing. Make things cheap, and they are almost sure to be despised. In our artificial state, we do not esteem things according to their real worth. And it is more than probable that hundreds, who now have as great an aversion to water as a mad dog has, would use it more fully, and would take more exercise in the open air, if these blessings were not also enjoyed by the working classes. This was not the case in England formerly; for Dr. Henry, in his "History of England," says, "The ancient Britons were noted for being swift of foot, having fine athletic frames, and great strength of body; their only drink was water." Mr. Raspail, in his twelve lectures on the physiology of health and disease, reported in the "Medical Times" of September 9, 1843, says, "In the state of nature, pure water is the best drink for every living being—the most delightful of all beverages." And the reason why it is not generally so regarded, is because we have departed from the simplicity of nature.

The celebrated John Wesley, that keen observer of men and things, published a work in 1747, called "Primitive Physic," (a most significant title) which has gone through near 100 editions, and is still extensively used. He recommends cold water internally and externally, both as a preventive and cure of disease. Webb, the noted pedestrian, remarkable for vigor of mind and body, was exclusively a water drinker. Cobbett, who in some respects was as great as he was singular, bears the following testimony to the benefit of water drinking, mentally and physically. "In the midst of a society, where wine and spirit are considered as of little more value than water, I have lived two years without either; and with no drink but water, except when I have found it convenient to obtain milk; not an hour's illness; not a headache for an hour; nor the smallest ailment; not a restless night; not a drowsy morning have I known during these two famous years of my life. The sun never rises before me; I have always to wait for him to come and give me light to write by, while my mind is full of vigor, and while nothing has come to cloud its clearness."

These united testimonies go to confirm all that has been said in praise of cold water—and show that it is, as has been often asserted, the grand beverage of organized nature, the drink appointed by a merciful and unerring God, to primeval man, and all attempts to improve it by the admixture of alcoholic, narcotic, or aromatic substances have only tended to injure or poison it, and those who have thus used it. The art of preparing liquors is the greatest curse ever inflicted on humanity. Water, which nature has so abundantly provided, is the best fitted for man to drink: it is suitable for every variety of constitution, and is more effectual than any other in allaying thirst, thereby showing it to be the beverage designed to supply the loss of fluids, to which we are perpetually subject. Simple aqueous drinks promote digestion, by facilitating the solution of solids, and by serving as a vehicle to their divided parts. The purest water is rendered stimulating by the air and salts it contains.—*Richerand.* (See Appendix, L.)

Simple water without any addition, is the proper drink of mankind.—*Cullen.*

When taken fresh and cold it is the most wholesome drink, and the most grateful to those who are thirsty, whether they be sick or well. It quenches the thirst, cools the body, and thereby destroys acrimony; it often promotes sweat, expels noxious matters, resists putrefaction, aids digestion, and in fine, strengthens the stomach.—*Dr. Gregory.*

When men contented themselves with water, they had more

health and strength; and at this day, those who drink nothing but water, are more healthy and live longer.—*Dr. Duncan.*

Beyond all peradventure, water was the primitive—the original beverage, and it is the only fluid fitted for the ends appointed by nature. Happy had it been for the race of mankind if other mixed and artificial liquors had never been invented.—*Dr. Cheyne.*

Look at the horse, with every muscle of his body swelled from morning to night in the plough or team; does he make signs for spirits to enable him to clear the earth, or climb the hills? No; he requires nothing but cold water and substantial food.—*Dr. Rush.*

The moment we depart from water, we are left, not to the instinct of nature, but to an artificial taste. Under the guidance of the instinct God has implanted within us, we are safe, but as soon as we leave it we are in danger.—*Dr. Oliver.*

The water drinker glides tranquilly through life, without much exhilaration or depression, and escapes many diseases to which others are subject. They have short but vivid periods of rapture, and long intervals of gloom. The balance of enjoyment then turns decidedly in favor of the water drinker; and there is but little doubt but that every person might, gradually, or even pretty quickly, accustom himself to the aqueous beverage.—*Dr. Johnson.*

The intellectual excitement produced by other drinks, is more than counterbalanced by the subsequent depression; and ruin of health, and abbreviation of life are the ultimate results.—*Thrackray.*

The strength which they seem to impart is temporary and unnatural. It is a present energy purchased at the expense of future weakness.—*Dr. K. Greville.*

Man in ordinary health, like all other animals, requires not any such stimulant, and cannot be benefited by the habitual employment of any quantity of them, large or small, etc.—*Eighty Eminent Surgeons.*

I assert that they are in every instance, as articles of diet, pernicious, and as medicines, wholly unnecessary, etc.—*Dr. E. Johnson.* (See Appendix, M.)

Water is the most suitable drink for man, is best fitted to prolong life, and does not chill the ardor of genius. Demosthenes' sole drink was water.—*Zimmerman.*

If people would accustom themselves to drink water, they would be free from many diseases, such as tremblings, apoplexies, giddiness, pain in the head, gout, stone, dropsy, rheumatism, and such like.—*Dr. Pratt.*

No remedy can more effectually secure health and prevent disease than pure water.—*Hoffman.*

Who has not observed the extreme satisfaction which children derive from quenching their thirst with pure water; and who that has perverted his appetite by beverages of human invention, but would be a gainer on the score of mere animal gratification, without any reference to health, if he would bring back his vitiated taste to the simple relish of nature.—*Dr. Oliver.*

Man is the only animal accustomed to swallow unnatural drink: water is the best diluent.—*Dr. Garnett.*

The healthy man requires only water.—*Dr. Farre.*

The best drink is water; a liquor commonly despised, and even by some people considered prejudicial; I will not hesitate, however, to declare it to be one of the greatest means of prolonging life: it is the greatest promoter of digestion, and by its coolness and fixed air, it is an excellent strengthener of the stomach and nerves.—*Dr. Hufeland.*

It is the chief ingredient in the animal fluids, and solids; for a dry bone distilled affords a quantity of insipid water; and the human brain is known to consist of more than eighty parts in every one hundred of water; therefore water appears to be the proper drink for every animal.—*Dr. Arbuthnot.*

It is my opinion, that those who belong to such a society (Nature's Beverage Society) will seldom have occasion for medical men.—*Dr. Orphen.*

Among other innumerable advantages which the water drinker enjoys, he saves a considerable sum of money per annum, which others waste in artificial drinks; and in drugs to cure the diseases which these drinks induce. The water drinker enjoys an exquisite sensibility of palate, and a relish for plain food that the wine drinker has no idea of. Happy those who are wise enough to be convinced that water is the best drink, and salt the best sauce.—*Dr. Kitchener.* (See Appendix, N.)

A multitude of other quotations might have been made, precisely of the same kind, from Sweetin, Bœerhave, Celsus, Cooper, Parr, Sydenham, Haller, Stahl, Hufeland, Galen, and Hippocrates, corroborated by 5000 medical men in America. Indeed, the experience of persons in all ages confirm the voice of God in nature, and in the Bible, that "all that drink water shall be comforted."

Mr. Priessnitz is of opinion that all persons may drink water without the slightest risk, in any quantity, only observing one rule: viz., never to drink so much as to be inconvenienced by it; and after a little practice, you will be able to determine how much you can take with advantage. The general rule should be about from twelve to thirty glasses per day. The patient should cease drinking, for the time, when it produces shivering, and should produce reaction by exertion. Dr. Wilson tells us, that when he was at Graefenburg, in eight months he took 500 cold baths, 400 sitz baths, and reposed 480 hours in a wet sheet, and drank about 3500 tumblers of cold water. He drank upward of thirty glasses one morning before breakfast,* and meant to have taken a few more, but was so hungry he could stay no longer. On some persons, drinking water produces diarrhœa, which, though it alarms them, proves to those who understand the mode of its operation, that it has disturbed bad humors which were lodged in the stomach, and

* Campbell, in his Travels in Africa, speaking of a Mr. Camver, who dined with him and his companions in their tent, says, he can drink nothing but water: indeed he is the greatest water drinker he ever heard of. I saw him drink three pints of water at supper the preceding evening, and he assured us he drank a pailful always during the night.

shows the propriety of continuing and even increasing its use. All times of the day are proper for drinking water, but the morning before breakfast is the best, especially if taken with exercise in the open air, as this stimulates the action of the water. It should be always taken fresh from its source and as cold as possible. If you have not the convenience of a good spring or pump to which you can repair, keep your water in a decanter, having a good stopper, in which it will remain longer cold, and preserve its fixed air. Much as water may be despised through our ignorance of its value, it is the only fluid provided by the Creator for the drink of innumerable animated beings who inhabit every part of the air, the earth, and the seas; and hence it might be reasonably inferred, that it is an agent in the promotion of health, strength, and longevity, of incalculable value. After many experiments, botanists have found that the cow eats of 276 kinds of grass and herbs; the horse of 262; the goat of 449; sheep of 387; and swine of only 72. But though deriving their nourishment from these various kinds of solid food, water is their only diluent (excepting the filthy hog),* the only one provided to quench their thirst, for cooling the fever to which they are occasionally subject, and for repairing the waste of the circulating fluids. Water alone as a drink is necessary to maintain the courage and strength of the lion, and the bulk and sagacity of the elephant. The bear, while roaming amidst icebergs, and the camel, while traveling over burning sands, and beneath a burning sky, have no other drink to protect them from the effects of cold in the one case, and of heat in the other. It is one of the greatest blessings bestowed upon man: "the Deity is the manufacturer; the ocean the raw material; the sun the genera-

* Whitlaw says, of all the abominable feeding creatures the swine may be said to be the chief; it is more liable to disease, and entails more misery on the human race than any other animal; we think with him, it would be no loss to man, if the whole breed of them had shared the fate of the Gadarean herd. Eating swine's flesh is the cause of most of our cutaneous diseases.

tor of the vapor ; the sky the condenser; electricity and attraction the distributors, in showers and dews, so finely attenuated as to be respired through the pores of the most delicate plants; rivers and lakes are so abundantly distributed as to support, not only the whole vegetable, but also the animal creation. It checks and extinguishes the most destructive ailments, and finds its level between the tops of mountains, and the tops of houses. It wants neither steamboat or locomotive to be transported. It cleanses and beautifies all nature, and is so salubrious to man, that it neither disorders the stomach, excites the passions, or maddens the brain: it is so necessary to all life that the humblest insect exists not without it. The loftiest monarch of the forest, and man the monarch of all, in its absence, drop their heads on the parched ground and die. In allusion to its cheering and refreshing virtues, the sacred record says, "As cold water to a thirsty soul, so is good news from a far country." It is made a grand emblem of greater blessings: hence, says Jehovah, "I will pour water upon him that is thirsty, and floods upon the dry ground." It was a "bottle of water" that Abraham gave to his handmaid Hagar to drink, when he sent her away from his dwelling; it was water with which the Almighty supplied her in the desert, and by which he graciously preserved her son Ishmael from death. When God engaged to supply the wants of his faithful ones by the prophet Isaiah, it is not luxuries that he promises, but simply "bread and water." Isaiah xxxiii. 16. A similar, but enlarged promise was given to the children of Israel in the days of Moses. Exodus xxiii. 25. When God threatened the Jews, in Isaiah iii. 1, it was to take away their "whole stay of bread and the whole stay of water." It was water that Elijah asked of the widow of Zarephath, and that was provided for him by the angel. We read of the well of which Jacob drank, and his children, and his cattle; and when the children of Israel in their journeys through the wilderness, were fed with bread from heaven, God, who could have given them wine, ale, tea, etc., had it been better for them, gave them water from the rock. And among the chief blessings of the land of Canaan, they were told by Moses it was "a land of brooks of water, of fountains and depths of water that spring out of the valleys and hills." The mighty Sampson was a water drinker, and when ready to faint, "God clave a hollow place in the jaw bone (his weapon with which he smote the Philistines), and there came water thereout, and when he had drank, his spirit came again, and he revived." Elijah drank of the brook Cherith, and Obadiah fed the prophets of the Lord with bread and water. Among the offences which Eliphaz unjustly charged upon Job, we find him saying: "Thou hast not given water to the weary to drink;" and as a striking illustration of the invigorating nature of water, the prophet Isaiah speaks of the smith while working at the forge as fainting for want of it. God himself is called "the Fountain of living water," as is also the enjoyment of the redeemed in glory.

The following verses are copied from the "Metropolitan Magazine," and form a happy contrast to the bacchanalian songs so frequently inserted in different journals:

SONG OF THE HOREBITE.

O! WATER for me! bright water for me,
And wine for the tremulous debauchee!
It cooleth the brow, it cooleth the brain,
It maketh the faint one strong again;
It comes o'er the sense like a breeze from the sea,
All freshness, like infant purity.
Oh! water, bright water for me, for me!
Give wine, give wine, to the debauchee!

Fill to the brim! fill, fill to the brim!
Let the flowing crystal kiss the rim!
For my hand is steady, my eye is true;
For I, like the flowers, drink nought but dew.
Oh! water, bright water's a mine of wealth,
And the ores it yieldeth are vigor and health.
So water, pure water for me, for me!
And wine for the tremulous debauchee!

Fill again to the brim! again to the brim!
For water strengtheneth life and limb!
To the days of the aged it addeth length,
To the might of the strong it addeth strength.
It freshens the heart, it brightens the sight,
'Tis like quaffing a goblet of morning light.
So water, I will drink nought but thee,
Thou parent of health and energy!

When o'er the hills, like a gladsome bride,
Morning walks forth in her beauty's pride,
And leading a band of laughing hours,
Brushes the dew from the nodding flowers;
Oh! cheerily then my voice is heard,
Mingling with that of the soaring bird,
As he freshens his wing in the cold grey cloud;

But when evening has quitted her sheltering yew,
Drowsily flying and weaving anew
Her dusky meshes o'er land and sea—
How gently, O sleep, fall thy poppies on me!
For I drink water, pure, cold, and bright,
And my dreams are of heaven the livelong night;
So hurrah for thee, water! Hurrah, hurrah!
Thou art silver and gold, thou art ribbon and star!
Hurrah for bright water! Hurrah, hurrah!—E. Johnson.

The disciples of the pump will hardly require an apology from us for presenting them with the following beautiful speech of our *one-armed friend,* slightly altered and abridged from the "New England Magazine."

[*Scene.*—The corner of two principal streets. The Town Pump talking through its nose.]

"Noon by the north clock! Noon by the east! High noon, too, by the hot sunbeams, which fall scarcely aslope upon my head, and almost make the water bubble and smoke in the trough under my nose. Truly, we public characters have a rough time of it! Among all the town officers, who sustains, for a single year, the burden of such manifold duties as are imposed in perpetuity upon the Town Pump? The title of town treasurer is rightfully mine; and as guardian of the best treasure the town has, the overseers of the poor ought to make me their chairman, since I provide bountifully to the pauper, without expense to the ratepayer. I am at the head of the fire department, and one of the physicians of the board of health. As a keeper of the peace, all water drinkers will confess me equal to the constable. I perform some of the duties of the town clerk, by promulgating public notices, when pasted on my front. To speak within bounds, I am chief person of the municipality, and exhibit an admirable pattern to my brother officers, by the cool, steady, upright, downright, and impartial discharge of my duties, and the constancy with which I stand at my post. . Summer or winter, nobody seeks me in vain; for, all day long, I am seen at the busiest corner, just above the market, stretching out my arm to rich and poor alike; and at night I hold a lantern over my head, both to show where I am and keep people out of the gutters. At this sultry noontide, I am cupbearer to the parched populace, for whose benefit an iron goblet is chained to my waist. I cry aloud to all and sundry in my plainest accents, and at the very tiptop of my voice, Here it is, gentlemen! here is the good liquor! Walk up, walk up, gentlemen, walk up, walk up! Here is the superior stuff! Here is the *unadulterated ale of father Adam*—better than Cognac, Hollands, Jamaica, strong beer, wine, tea, coffee, or cocoa! Here it is by the hogshead or the glass, and not a farthing to pay! Walk up, gentlemen, and help your selves! It were a pity if all this outcry should draw no customers. Here they come. A hot day, gentlemen, quaff, and away again, so as to keep yourselves in a nice cool sweat. You, my friend, will need another cupful to wash the dust out of your throat, if it be as thick there as it is on your shoes. I see you have trudged half-a-score miles to-day, and, a wise man, have passed by the taverns, and stopped at the running brooks. Otherwise, betwixt heat without and fire within, you would have been burnt to a cinder, or melted down to nothing at all, in the fashion of a jelly-fish. Drink, and make room for that fellow who seeks my aid to quench the fiery fever of last night's potations, which he drained from no cup of mine. Welcome, most rubicund sir! You and I have been great strangers, hitherto; nor, to confess the truth, will my nose be anxious for a closer intimacy, till the fumes of your breath be a little less potent. Mercy on you, man! The water absolutely hisses down your red-hot gullet, and is converted quite into steam in the miniature Tophet which you mistake for a stomach. Fill again, and tell me, did you ever, in beer-shop, tavern, or dram-shop, spend the price of your children's food for a swig half so delicious? Now, for the first time these ten years, you know the flavor of cold water. Good bye! and whenever you are thirsty, remember that I keep a constant supply at the old stand. What next! Oh, my little friend, you are let loose from school, and come here to scrub your blooming face, and drown the memory of certain taps of the ferule, and other schoolboy troubles; take it, and may your heart and tongue never be scorched with a fiercer thirst than now! There, my dear, put down the cup, and yield your place to this elderly gentleman, who treads so tenderly over the paving stones, that I suspect he is afraid of breaking them. What! He limps by, without so much as thanking me, as if my hospitable offers were only meant for people who have no wine-cellars. Well, well, sir, no harm done, I hope! Go, draw the cork, tip the decanter; but when your great toe shall set you a-roaring, it will be no affair of mine. If gentlemen love the pleasant titillation of the gout, it is all one to the Town Pump. This thirsty dog, with his red tongue lolling out, does not scorn my hospitality, but stands on his hind legs and laps eagerly out of the trough. See how lightly he capers away again. Jowler, had you ever the gout? Then wipe your mouths, my good friends; and while my spout has a moment's leisure, I will delight you with a few historical reminiscences. In far-famed antiquity, beneath a darksome shadow of venerable boughs, a spring bubbled out of the leaf-strewn earth, in the very spot where you now behold me on the sunny pavement.

The water was as bright and clear, and deemed as precious, as liquid diamonds. Your primitive forefathers drank of it from time immemorial, when the art of preparing the *accursed draught* was unknown in the land. The young and grayheaded often knelt down on the grass beside the spring, and drank of its cool and refreshing stream. For many years it was the watering-place, and, as it were, the washbowl of the vicinity, whither all decent folks resorted to purify their visages, and gaze—at least the pretty maidens did—in the mirror it made. On Sabbath days, whenever a babe was to be baptized, the sexton filled his basin here, and placed it on the communion-table of the humble church, which partly covered the sight of yonder stately edifice. Thus one generation after another was consecrated to Heaven by its waters, and cast their waxing and waning shadows into its glassy bosom, and vanished from the earth, as if mortal life were but a flitting image in a fountain! Finally, the fountain vanished also; cellars were dug on all sides, and cartloads of gravel were flung upon its source, whence oozed a turpid stream, forming a puddle in the corner of two streets. In the hot months, when its refreshment was most needed, the dust flew in clouds over the forgotten birth-place of the waters, now their grave. But in the course of time a Town Pump was sunk into the source of its ancient spring. When the first decayed, another took its place, then another, and still another—till here I stand, ladies and gentlemen, to serve you. Drink and be refreshed! The water is as pure and cold as that which slaked the thirst of your venerable ancestors, beneath the aged boughs, though now the gem of the wilderness is treasured under these hot stones, where no shadow falls but from the brick buildings. And be it the moral of my story, that as *this wasted and long-lost fountain is now known and prized again, so shall the virtues of cold water, too little valued since our father's days, be yet recognized by all.* Your pardon, good people! I must interrupt my stream of eloquence, and spout forth a stream of water, to replenish the trough for this drover and his oxen, who have come from afar.

No part of my business is pleasanter than the watering of cattle. Look how rapidly they lower the water-mark on the sides of the trough, till their capacious stomachs are moistened with a gallon or two a-piece, and they can afford time to breathe it in with sighs of calm enjoyment. Now they roll their quiet eyes around the rim of their monstrous drinking vessel. An ox is your true toper. But I perceive, my dear auditors, that you are impatient for the remainder of my discourse. Impute it, I beseech you, to no defect of modesty, if I insist a little longer on so fruitful a topic as my own multifarious merits. It is altogether for your good. The better you think of me the better men and women you will find yourselves. I shall say nothing of my all-important aid on washing-days, though on that account alone I might call myself the household-god of a hundred families. Far be it from me, also, to hint at the show of dirty faces which you would present without my pains to keep you clean. Nor will I remind you how often, when the midnight bells made you tremble for your combustible town, you fled to the Town Pump, and found me always at my post, firm amid the confusion, and ready to drain my vital current on your behalf; neither is it worth while to lay undue stress on my claims to a medical diploma, as the physician whose simple rule of practice is preferable to all the nauseous lore which has found men sick or left them so, since the days of Hippocrates. Let us take a broader view of my beneficial influence on mankind. No, these are trifles, compared with the merits which wise men concede to me, if not in my single self, yet as the representative of a class—of being the *grand reformer of the age*. From my spout, and such spouts as mine, must flow the stream that shall cleanse our earth of a vast portion of its crime and anguish, which has gushed from the fiery fountains of the still and the beer vat. In this mighty enterprise the cow shall be my great confederate. Water and milk! The Town Pump and the cow! Such is the glorious copartnership that shall tear down the distilleries, brew-houses, and malt-kilns, and finally monopolize the whole business of quenching thirst. Blessed consummation! When shall the glorious day dawn upon us!

"Ahem! dry work, this speechifying' especially to an unpracticed orator. I never conceived, till now, what toil the temperance lecturers undergo for my sake. Hereafter they shall have the business to themselves. Do, some kind Christians, pump a stroke or two, just to wet my whistle! Thank you, sir! My dear hearers, by my instrumentality you will collect your useless vats, liquor-casks, and beer-barrels into one great pile, and make a bonfire, in honor of the Town Pump; and when I shall have decayed, like my predecessors, then, if you revere my memory, let a marble fountain, richly sculptured, take my place upon this spot. Such monuments should be erected every where, and inscribed with the names of the distinguished champions of my cause. There are some honest and true friends of mine, who, nevertheless, by their fiery pugnacity in my behalf, do put me in fearful hazard of a broken nose, or even of a total overthrow upon the pavement, and the loss of the treasure which I guard. I pray you, gentlemen, let this fault be amended. In the moral warfare which you are to wage, and indeed in the whole conduct of your lives, you cannot choose a better example than myself, who has never permitted the dust and sultry atmosphere, the turbulence and manifold disquietudes of the world around us, to reach that deep, calm well of purity, which may be called my soul; and whenever I pour out that soul, it is to cool earth's fevers, or to wash its stains. One o'clock! Nay, then, if the dinner-bell begins to speak, I may as well hold my peace. Here comes a pretty young girl of my acquaintance, with a large stone pitcher for me to fill. May she draw a husband, while drawing her water, as Rachel did of old! Hold out your vessel, my dear! There, it is full to the brim; so now run home, peeping at your sweet image in the pitcher as you go, and forget not, in a glass of my own liquor, to drink, 'Success to the Town Pump!'" When the happy day shall arrive that the banded sons of temperance shall fully carry out their principles; when they shall abandon all artificial drinks, and become, indeed, water drinkers, then their wives, their sons, and their daughters, and the banners around which they shall rally, for the life of the nations, and the elevation of their own characters, shall shine forth with wisdom's mottos—"All that drink water shall be comforted!" "No distillation but the dew of heaven!" "No drink but the crystal well!" When the voice of the whole people shall go forth, saying, "Let the golden grain be all gathered to our garners, and let man feed on the fat of the land; let the land be occupied in growing useful vegetables and herbs, roots, and fruit, and not useless tea, coffee, etc.; let the fruit of the trees ripen only to give sweetening and variety to man's necessary food, and let none forsake their own mercies for useless and injurious articles, which give not strength to the system, but only tend to pamper a vitiated appetite; let them come to vegetable diet and water;" then shall every cheek glow with health, man's life be greatly lengthened, his enjoyments vastly increased, and his labor and anxiety much diminished. Sleep shall be sweet to the weary, and joy again be in the habitation of woe. Love and peace shall prevail, and the blessings of cold water and vegetable food enhance the value of every other earthly blessing. When the dayspring from on high shall visit us, and the pure water of life flow as a river, to purify and refresh the soul, then shall the earth bring forth her increase, and God, even our God, shall bless us; then, ye favored sons and daughters of Britain, whose heritage this may be, with all the most benign gifts of God "whatsoever things are pure, whatsoever things are lovely, whatsoever things are of good report; if there be any virtue, if there be any praise, think on these things."

After nearly three years' abstinence from all artificial drink, the increase of health, and vigor of body and mind, and the return of a natural appetite, which enables its possessor to enjoy plain food, we bid farewell to all but nature's beverage; and while some are quaffing strong drinks, scalding tea, etc., and fancying they should be greatly abridging their comforts if they were to abandon them, every member of Nature's Beverage Society exclaims, "Give me reviving and purifying water! the rills, the stream, or the torrent which pours from the bright sides of our cloud-crested mountains; the gush, cool and clear, that bubbled up before Hagar and the fainting Ishmael; that followed the stroke of the prophet's rod, from the rock of Horeb; that refreshed the inhabitants of Paradise! Give me the pure water that Isaac drank from the pitcher of Rebekah; that Elijah received from the hand of the angel, and the Saviour enjoyed at the well of Jacob; that cheered the spirits of the favored Israelites, the valiant Gideonites, the noble Nazarites, and the honored Rechabites; that quenched the thirst of mighty Samson, the holy Daniel, the fearless John, and the youthful Timothy! Give me of these cheering springs, these flowing brooks, and these crystal rivers, whose transparent surface reflects all that is calm, or soft, or bright in the beautiful firmament above! Give me those gentle streams, in health and in sickness; give me those waters, untainted and free, until I drink of that river, 'the streams whereof make glad the city of our God.'"

PART III.

CHAPTER VIII.

ON DRUGS.

Thus with our hellish drugs, death's ceaseless fountains,
In these bright vales, o'er these green mountains,
Worse than the very plague we raged.
I have myself to thousands poison given,
And heard their murderer praised as blest by Heaven,
Because with nature strife he waged. GOETHE'S FAUST

There has been a great increase of medical men, it is true, of late years; but, upon my life, diseases have increased in proportion.—ABERNETHY'S SURGICAL LECTURES.

PREVENTION is better than cure.* It must, therefore, be of more importance to know how to preserve health, than to be able to find out the cause which has deprived them of it, or the means which promote its restoration. To accomplish this, however, we must not depend on others, no, not even on the "Faculty;"† but we must employ the capabilities within

* Dr. Cheyne observes, most men know when they are ill, but very few when they are well. And yet it is certain that it is easier to preserve health than to recover it, and to prevent diseases than to cure them. Toward the first, the means are mostly in our own power; little less is required than to bear and forbear. But toward the latter the means are perplexing and uncertain. Yet nothing is more common with the short-sighted victims of disease, than to prefer palliating their torments by drugs, to preventing them by proper regimen; and you may as well try to reason with a mad dog as with some of these, although an experiment of six months would forever set the question at rest.

† Dr. Dickson has written an admirable and philosophic work on the "Fallacy of the Faculty," in which he says, "Until mankind cease to

our own reach. We have been looking for help from others too long; and it is a melancholy fact that, independent of multitudes who are swept off the stage of life in spite of, or, in some instances, in consequence of the host of physicians, surgeons, druggists, etc., who are well paid* to preserve the public health, scarcely has a man reached his fortieth year before he feels he is grown old and decrepit—a proof that we cannot depend upon the faculty. Nor is it all necessary, seeing "this is not a matter of speculative science, nor of normal art; but a matter simply and exclusively of common sense."

prefer signs to sense, men's words to the examination of God's works; until they take the trouble to make themselves acquainted with the laws of their own economy, they never can learn to distinguish the true physician from the mere pretender, whether the latter be a literate person with a diploma, or an unlettered quack without it."

* Could we get a correct account of the sums spent annually in drugs, hospitals, madhouses, doctors, etc., we should be astounded. [Think of the princely wealth, amassed by patent-medicine venders, and of the pill-warehouses in London, like castles. It is a fact, which we can state upon excellent authority, that one house in London shipped six tons of blue pills, at once, for South America.] It is not so in other countries, showing that there is something wrong in our "state of Denmark." In China, for instance, there are no surgeons at all: nature and temperance do for them more than all our doctors and drugs can do for us. Perhaps one principal reason why their physicians are so successful, though not half so learned as ours, is because—no cure, no pay. And is not this rational? Is it not calculated to make it the interest of medical men to exert their skill in curing their patients quickly? We pay for physic what we deny for talent; for a long illness what we refuse to speedy recovery; as if we thought medical men, above all others, were incapable of being influenced by temptation, while our very mode of remunerating them forces them to be corrupt. We do this, too, at a time when their numbers are so great that, could even one half of them live honestly, the other half must starve. What a happy nation of fools must that be, which supposes that any class of mankind will put the interests of the public in competition with their own! This is not the rule, but the exception, and is only found where grace has implanted it. Disinterested benevolence is an exotic, and its possessor is born from above—is a new creature, and therefore can do exploits of which poor human nature is utterly incapable.

There is great reason, we think, to endeavor to open the eyes of the public, as to the evils of the present mode of doing business, on accornt of the little dependence that can be placed on the opinions of medical men, and the small amount of relief that can be expected from drugs, themselves being judges: for, as Dr. Harrison justly observes, "I need not tell you," who have made this a subject of investigation, "that there are very few diseases for which we have nearly certain cures; that the use of remedies of great and general efficacy, for the cure of particular diseases, is at least precarious, often unavailing, and sometimes pernicious. In consequence of this imperfect state of medicine, vast multitudes every year languish long, at last die of consumption, dropsy, gout, stone, king's-evil, cancer, asthma, etc., etc., in spite of all our faculty can do for them." There are thousands of persons who have so debilitated their constitutions by departing from nature's laws, that though they are daily proving in their own persons the truth of Dr. Harrison's remarks, yet are so blinded by, and prejudiced in favor of, the old system, that they think they are among the "millions in this country to whom," Dr. Johnson says, "physic is daily as indispensable as food."* These people will not believe their own senses,† and

* I am sure I am within the bounding of truth, when I assert, that, throughout England, there is not more than one man in a hundred who does not find it necessary, at least once a month, to take medicine; that is, to carry the masterpiece of God's creative wisdom to the doctor, to have it mended. Why, I would discard my tinker if my saucepan required mending so often.—*Dr. E. Johnson.*

† This reminds us of a story told of an Irish sailor in a naval fight, who was commanded to clear the decks, preparatory to a second engagement with the enemy's vessel. The dead were to be thrown overboard, while the wounded were carried below. Of course the doctor went round to see where life was extinct; but in one instance in which he pronounced the man as dead, the poor fellow had only fainted. The sailor went on with his work, casting one with another overboard, until at last he came to the man who had fainted, and who was just coming to himself. The sailor was about to cast him overboard, when he faintly said, "I am not dead." This was a fact; but the sailor was like many more now in ref-

would be even more indignant than the doctors themselves, if the plan of Dr. Forth was acted upon in this country. He asserts that, "a monarch who could free his state from this pestilent set of physicians and apothecaries, and entirely interdict the practice of medicine, would deserve to be placed by the side of the most illustrious characters who have ever conferred benefits on mankind. There is scarcely a more dishonest trade* imaginable than that of medicine in its present state." Mr Whitlaw says, "I most anxiously pray that the physical leaders of this great empire may pause before it is too late, and no longer humbug the people by tracing out effects without a cause, which is the greatest insult to God's moral government of the universe, as the whole of his works are cause and effect." (See Appendix, O.)

Perhaps few circumstances have tended more to create suspicion in the minds of the thinking portion of the community, as to the "fallacy of the faculty," than the ambiguous manner and dark phraseology† by which medical men have expressed

erence to drugs—he preferred authority to fact—and exclaimed, "Arrah now, nonsense, not dead! The doctor says you are dead, and he knows better than you!" So we urge the fact that, notwithstanding the public have been drenched with drugs, and have gone on in a course of physical degeneracy, it is all to no purpose—authority is their reason, and to the voice of common sense, and living facts, they cry—"Arrah, nonsense! man must be a diseased creature—he must die early—he cannot do without medicine—the doctor says so, and he knows better than we do." See "British Temperance Advocate."

* Physicians in despair of making medicine a science, have agreed to convert it into a trade.—*Dr. Akenside.*

† A medical witness being examined at the Old Bailey, on a case before the court, used the word tumefaction; upon which Mr. Justice Coleridge said, "I suppose by tumefaction, you mean swelling?" Witness: "Yes, my lord," Mr. Coleridge: "Then would it not be much better to use plain English than to speak in a sort of mongrel Latin?" We say, yes, my lord; better for the health and pockets of the people, but not for keeping up the farce of drugging and fleecing them; for, as held by Dr. Kitchener, and the celebrated Dr. J. Brown, "If medicine be entirely divested of its mystery, its power over the mind, which in most cases forms its main strength, will no longer exist."

themselves. In general, who among the uninitiated think of reading medical works? Or, if they should attempt it, do they not find it absolutely necessary to have a medical dictionary at their elbow? Who thinks of asking his medical attendant why he recommends such a course to his patient? "Give reasons, indeed! no, not if they were as plentiful as blackberries in autumn." Porter, ale, spirits, drugs, etc., have been administered in profusion, when it would have occasioned great uneasiness if a reason had been sought to justify the practice, simply because that is a scarce commodity with most practitioners, they having imbibed "their creed in the surgery of their master." They believe "that mercury* is good in liver complaints, and is to be tried in all complaints, when all other remedies have failed; that purgatives are always demanded; that bleeding, opiates, and emetic sudorifics are fit for rheumatism; that colchicum defieth gout; that sal volatile, valerian, and sundry other ill-flavored stuffs, are requisite for hysterical women; that indigestion—that puzzling protean fiend—is to be combated pell-mell by all the above remedies."

According to this mode of doing business, what does it matter whether a man be well versed in medical science, or be a mere novice; he can easily proceed in the old beaten track, because "the remedies are named opposite the disease; nay more, there are remedies to counteract the evil effects of other remedies.† 'Acts to amend certain acts passed' in the last

* In Holland, physicians are prosecuted and heavily fined for administering mercury. There are few chemists' shops there; and since the law has prohibited the administration of mercury, disease has greatly decreased.

† I lately met with a country practitioner, who, upon being asked by a lady whom he attended, the intention of three different draughts which he had sent her, replied that one would warm, the second cool her, and the third was calculated to moderate the too violent effects of either. The same doctor (Paris) remarks: "The file of every apothecary would furnish a volume of instances where the ingredients of the prescription are fighting together in the dark, or at least, are so adverse to each other, as to constitute a most incongruous and chaotic mass."

prescription. Moreover, the remedies are known to themselves; unknown to their patients, whose queries, if any, are answered in an unknown tongue of technicality. The whole process, in fact, is one of jog-trot routine, whereby if the patient recovers, *so*—he must take some tonics; if he dies, *so*—he swallowed the pharmacopœia, and what can a man do more?"—*Drs. Wilson and Gully.* To such inquiries we say, why, if you must continue in practice, study its philosophy, that you may be able to give the people scientific truth in exchange for their cash, and a plain, straightforward "answer to every man who asketh you a reason of the hope" you entertain of the efficacy of your mode of treatment; and not in the "pretty gibberish invented to cheat the ignorant," and to mystify your practice. Who has not been placed in a similar position to that of the person to whom Dr. E. Johnson wrote those admirable letters on "Life, Health, and Disease?" He had been for some time laboring under a "combination of most dissimilar symptoms, all of which, he was assured, are presented by the term indigestion." When he questioned his medical attendants on the subject, they evinced every disposition to satisfy him; but they could not avoid making use of phrases which were to him words without meaning. He was told that his digestion was impaired. He asked what was meant by that, and was told his "digestive apparatus was deranged in its economy." My poor brother was still no nearer the mark; and his medical attendant observing his puzzled looks, proceeded to explain and make the matter perfectly clear, telling him that his "secretions were depraved, his gastric juices deficient, his native functions feebly performed, and that the tone, the energy, the nisus formatives—in fact, the vis vitæ—was full twenty per cent. below par." The enlightened patient bowed his gratitude for this luminous explanation, and sadly reseated himself in his chair of sickness—as wise, perhaps, but certainly no wiser, than he was before. How should he? There was nothing in all this likely to convey any definite idea to his mind, as to the nature or cause of the evil under which he was laboring, or the proper means of removing it. His medical attendant was to him, what St. Paul (1 Cor. xiv. 11) calls a barbarian, speaking in an unknown tongue. This is a very proper term, applicable to all who, while they articulate sounds, convey thereby no distinct meaning to their hearers. This is not learning, as it is thought to be by some, but barbarism: or, in the language of Horne Tooke, "an example of the subtle art of saving appearances, and of discoursing learnedly on a subject with which we are perfectly unacquainted." For instance, if you ask one of those learned gentlemen, "why opium sets you to sleep," his answer will be, "from its narcotic power. Narcotic comes from the Greek word narcosis, privation of sense." How satisfactory! Now those who are weak enough to believe all that is told them, whether they understand it or not, are delighted to be told in Greek that it does set them to sleep. *They* are astonished, and *he* is a very learned man. Thus they

> "Wrap nonsense round
> In pomp and darkness, till it seems profound;
> Play on the hopes, the terrors of mankind
> With changeful skill; * * * *
> While reason, like a grave-face mummy, stands
> With her arms swathed in hieroglyphic bands."—*Moore.*

Such is the mode in which the schoolmen juggle: instead of an answer they give you an echo! Had these barbarian wordmongers been as anxious to enlighten the public mind as they have been to feather their own nests, they would, long ago, have preferred reason to mystification, and thus advanced the good of the community at large.* But as the great Locke justly observes, "Vague and insignificant forms of speech, and abuse of language, have so long passed for mysteries of science, and hard and misapplied words, with little or no meaning, have, by prescription, such a right to be mistaken for deep

* See much on this subject in that withering exposé of the faculty by Dr. Dickson, of which he has published a "People's Edition."

learning and height of speculation, that it will not be easy to persuade either those who speak or those who hear them, that they are but the covers of ignorance and hindrances of true knowledge."

In consequence of the obscure language commonly employed by the faculty, the people have been deterred from investigating a subject, in which, of all others, they are most deeply and intimately concerned. But as most other antiquated notions and systems are being weighed in the even-handed balances of an enlightened people, and many of them have been "found wanting," is it any wonder that the drug system should be submitted to the analysis of common sense? The introduction of steam, galvanism, gas, etc., have produced a revolution of thought and action; petty objects have given way to comprehensive views; and petty interests have been made to yield to the general good, by the force of the no-monopoly principle. Is the drugging system to claim an exemption? On what ground? Let the protectionists tell us.

We are far from being satisfied with our hydropathic doctors. There is evidently, in some of them, a disposition to retain two of the old evils—monopoly and high charges; the latter they seek to accomplish by means of the former. (See Appendix, P.) If they realize their object, the poor especially will be prevented from enjoying the benefit of the water cure, in case of accident, etc. They cannot pay £3 per week, while in one of the establishments, besides traveling expenses and loss of time, etc. And because a few benevolent individuals have tried, partially, to remedy the evil, they have been denounced. Well, be it so. Let them persevere, and they will live down such interested opposition, and be regarded as the benefactors of their race when their traducers are covered with merited disgrace. The makers and venders of strong drinks, swords, drugs, tea, Jack Ketch, the grave-digger, etc., like these, have adopted the old, but ruinous maxim—"Live and let live." This is utterly impossible. How can they live if others persist in living also.

Though we place little confidence in the opinions of the advocates of drugs, the public does; and as in most cases, the best way to get at the whole truth, is, if possible, to hear the statements of those who have been "behind the scene," we shall avail ourselves of the views of a few of the initiated. It would, however, be an endless task, and produce an evil we are anxious to avoid (a large book), to quote all the just sarcasms and severe criticisms of medical men of high repute on their own profession, many of whom confessed they were skeptics in the science, and, as a proof of their sincerity, they beat their lancets into ploughshares, and left the profession in disgust. Among others, we mention Sir James Mackintosh, Locke, Crabbe, M'Kenzie, Sir H. Davy, and Lord Longdale.

Sir W. Knighton, who was at the head of his profession, and was also physician to George IV., says, "It is somewhat strange that though in many arts and sciences improvement has advanced in a step of regular progression from the first, in others it has kept no pace with time; and we look back to ancient excellence with wonder not unmixed with awe. Medicine seems to be one of those ill-fated arts whose improvement bears no proportion to its antiquity."

Had not facts borne out the truth of the doctor's statement, how could we account for the fact, that there has been, as Mr. Abernethy observes, an increase of disease; nay, many new ones, of only three or four hundred years' standing. Some even less than that—diseases quite unknown to the ancients. Measles is a complaint of modern times; scarlatina still more recent, having made its appearance only about two hundred years ago. The small-pox is of no very ancient date, since Hippocrates, Galen, etc., give it no place in their nosological histories. We learn from "Barrow's Travels," that to this day, Southern Africa is wholly exempt from small-pox and canine madness. It seems no writer mentions scurvy before Strabo, who tells us that it broke out for the first time in Augustus' reign, at which period we know how luxurious the Romans had become.

The celebrated Dr. J. Gregory, the leading physician of the city of Edinburgh, who held his profession in disgust, asserts, that medical doctrines are little better than stark staring absurdities. Being asked what he thought of Dr. Baillie, he replied, "Baillie knows nothing but physic;" in revenge for which, Baillie wittily rejoined, "Gregory knows every thing *but* physic." Dr. Dickson, says, "How I ever came to believe one half of the rubbish propounded by medical teachers, I cannot now understand ;-for the whole doctrine of the schools is a tissue of the most glaring and self-evident absurdities."—"Could you only see as I have seen," says Dr. Dickson, "the farce* of a medical consultation, I think you would agree with me, that the impersonification of physic, like the picture of Garrick, might be best painted with comedy on one side, and tragedy on the other." "Less slaughter, I am convinced, has been effected by the sword than by the lancet."† Again, "Of the cases of mortality in the earlier months of our existence, no small proportion consists of those who have sunk under the oppression of pharmaceutical filth. More infantile subjects in this metropolis, are, perhaps, diurnally destroyed by the mortar and pestle than in the ancient Bethlehem fell victims in one day to the Herodian massacre." And again, "Conscience feels little concern in cases of medicinal murder." This is "speaking out" with a vengeance, as the "racking effects of these days."

* The author recollects an instance which came under his own observation, some years ago, which greatly tended to shake his faith in druggery. An eminent physician of the city of Worcester being called in to his friend, who was living in a lone farmhouse, and where the author was visiting, after a few questions had been put and answered, the doctor, on examining the patient's pulse, held with his other hand his gold watch to his ear, for at least two minutes. Some general directions having been given, and a few compliments passed, the doctor was about to withdraw, when the lady of the house, informing him that her clock had stopped in the night, wished to know the city time, in order to set the clock right—when, lo! behold! the doctor discovered that his watch also had stopped in the night, he having forgotten to wind it up. How was it that the doctor did not discover this when counting the pulsations of his patient?

† Reid's Essays on Insanity

In the "British and Foreign Review," of January, 1838, we have the following testimony of one of the most eminent physicians of London. He says, "I visited the different schools, and the students of each other hinted, if they did not assert, that the other sects killed their patients. I found that, provided the physician of each was a man of talent and experience, the mortality was fairly balanced." The same "Review," speaking of the gentlemen in the chemical line, whose section of the business it is to supply the material of adulteration* to the brewers, etc., says, "Unless our information is very incorrect, there are not many prescriptions faithfully prepared in the British dominions. We believe there is scarcely a medicine, however simple, which the chemists' art cannot imitate, in cheap and base material; yet physicians prescribe with calm satisfaction." Dr. Franks asserts, that "thousands are slaughtered in the quiet sick-room."

It were easy to collect, from the pages of medical writers, of note in their day, numerous passages of similar import; but we pass on to give one or two from non-professional writers.

Voltaire gives an account of one Zadig, who, in an engagement, was dangerously wounded in the eye, near to which an

* Dr. Lardner says, "It is absolutely frightful to contemplate the list of poisons and drugs with which porter has been doctored." He mentions, among others, "opium, henbane, coculus indicus, aloes, and oil of vitriol;" and he might have added, tobacco, grains of paradise, saltpetre, nux vomica, etc. (See Appendix, Q.) From parliamentary returns, we find that some years the duty paid to government—

For nux vomica, was	£631	4*s*.	2*d*.
" extract of do., ...	4	7	6
" coculus indicus, ...	579	19	5
" grains of paradise, ...	3191	2	2

The consumption of these, which have been chiefly employed in making beer and porter, has, of late years, increased. Nux vomica, for example, which is a horrid poison, paid duty, in 1830, £191, but, in 1833, it paid £517 15*s*.; coculu[s i]ndicus, in 1829, £139 15*s*., but, in 1833, £569 19*s*. 5*d*. (See more i[n "] Bacchus," chap. xi., and "Anti-Bacchus," pp. 71, 72.)

abscess formed. The alarm became great, and Hermes, the celebrated physician, was sent for, who came, attended by a numerous retinue, and pronounced that Zadig would lose his eye, and even predicted the day and the hour when the dreadful accident would take place. Had it been the right eye, said he, I could have cured it; but the wounds of the left eye are without remedy. All Babylon, in deploring the fate of Zadig, venerated the profound knowledge of Hermes. Two days after, the tumor discharged itself spontaneously, and Zadig was perfectly cured. Hermes wrote a book, in which his object was to prove that Zadig ought not to have been cured.

Lord Byron called medicine "the destructive art of healing," and on one occasion says, "I got well [of a fever], by the blessing of barley water, and refusing to see my physician."*

Moliere, so long the terror of the apothecaries of Paris, makes one of his *dramatis personæ* say to another, "Call in a doctor, and if you do not like his physic, I'll soon find you another who will condemn it;" showing how completely at variance medical authorities are, so that perhaps it would be difficult to find any two of them agreeing. (See Appendix, R.) For proof of this, we refer our readers to the "Fallacy of the Faculty."

Le Sage was even more severe, when he said, "Death has two wings: on one are war, plague, famine, fire, shipwreck, with all the other miseries, that present him, at every instance, with a new prey; on the other wing you behold a crowd of young physicians, about to take their degrees before him. Death, with a demon smile, dubs them doctors, having first

* Some people tell you, with an air of the miraculous, that they recovered, although given over by their doctor; when they might, with more reason, have said, they recovered because they were given over. How just was the observation of the author of "Lacon:" "The rich patient cures the poor physician much oftener than the poor physician the rich patient; and the rapid recovery of the one usually depends upon the procrastinated disorder of the other."

made them swear never, in any way, to alter the established practice of physic."

Locke, Smollett, Goldsmith (all three physicians), held their art in contempt; Swift, Temple, Hume, Adam Smith, Hazlitt, etc., were equally severe.

That shrewd observer of human nature, John Wesley, published a work, in 1747, in which, after deprecating the mysteries with which the science of medicine is surrounded, and the manner in which drugs were imposed upon the community, he proceeds in a manner which shows that he thought water might very profitably supersede the use of drugs altogether. He says, "The common method of compounding and decompounding medicines can never be reconciled to common sense. Experience shows that one thing will cure most diseases, at least as well as twenty put together. Then why add the other nineteen? Only to swell the apothecary's bill; nay, possibly, on purpose to prolong the distemper, that the doctor and he may divide the spoil."

Captain Claridge, having inquired by what delusions mankind were first induced to take drugs, says, "In the middle ages, the use of water as a drink, and a cure for diseases, fell into total disuse, when, in the time of the Crusade, the Arabian doctors introduced the use of oriental drugs, to which they attributed miraculous virtues. But were these the dictates of reason and nature? Have mankind become healthier since their introduction? Quite the reverse! Are those nations, who have done the most homage to this science, the strongest and soundest? They are, beyond contradiction, physically, if not morally, the most miserable of all. How is it with individuals? Their lives are worse than death. Nay, even the masters of physic suffer very severely from its effects themselves." He further says, "This is the most dreadful malady of mankind; the poison-plague, dug out, by themselves, from the black abysses of the earth; thus has it been stared at as the effects of deep science, for centuries; thus has frequently the last shilling been offered at its altar. For this, the greatest enemy that could have beset mankind, as many millions have been spent as would pay off the national debt. To the study of these dangerous errors, have millions of men applied the whole of their lives and abilities. Backed by science, they contended against nature; but how does she punish those who wish to master her!"

This last quotation gives us a clue to the evil. The effects have been mistaken for the causes, and this error in judgment has led to errors in practice. For instance, as Constant justly observes, "It is now generally admitted, that many of the seemingly violent phenomena of inflammations are not, strictly speaking, morbid movements, but consist, in part at least, simply of energetic endeavors of nature to rid herself of an injurious agent or influence." The drugging system is at war with, in opposition to, nature—actually obstructing her operations. Hence, if nature seeks to relieve herself by vomiting, she is insulted by a dose of brandy; and in many cases, by these and other means, by violently increasing the vital force, it is ultimately destroyed. Whereas, the object should be, not to oppose but to assist nature, by placing the diseased organism generally on such a footing as shall enable their vegetative and conservative properties to operate as easily and as efficiently as possible; to develop their power, and compensate, by an act of self-reparation, for any disturbing influence of the morbid agent. This, in fact, is the object sought in the hydropathic mode of treatment, and is generally effected. This effect, however, is not produced so much by our measure, as by nature herself; and all that we can do is to liberate the normal action from any oppressing or obstructing causes, and afford it freedom of exertion.* In many cases—such as slight indigestion,

* Dr. Craigie, a popular writer, says: "When healthy properties are impaired, we know of no agent by which they can be directly restored; when vital action is perverted or deranged, we possess no means of immediately rectifying it, but must be satisfied with using those means under which it is most likely to rectify itself." This, we maintain, is a rational and common-sense view of the subject.

etc.—twenty-four hours' abstinence, or ceasing to load our already over-burdened stomach, with free exercise in the open air, and copious draughts of cold water, will render any other remedy altogether unnecessary. Some rather serious cases have come under our observation—such as vertigo, etc.—which have been cured by little else than putting the patient under proper regimen, allowing from nine to twelve ounces of bread, and from four to eight ounces of water per day, for several weeks. And we could produce high medical authority in support of the theory, that remedial means, no matter of what kind, possess in themselves no power of directly changing a diseased condition into a healthy one. All that it can effect is, to aid the efforts of the body in its own restoration; to accomplish which, we challenge drugs to a competition with water.

As successful results are the test of medical, as well as of all other truth, and is the professed aim of all treatment, we appeal to this tribunal, believing, with Dr. Macartney, one of the first physiologists of his day, that "water, when its properties and modes of application are well known, will be worth all other remedies put together." A conviction of this kind induced Bernardo, a monk of Sicily, in the year 1724, to go to Malta, where he effected some astonishing cures with water, the fame of which spread throughout Europe. The water was iced, which he used internally and externally. He allowed his patient to eat very little. The doctors laughed at him at first, but confident of the soundness of his theory, and of the superior efficacy of his plan to theirs, he made a proposition that they should take one hundred patients, and said if they, by their mode of treatment, could cure forty, he would undertake to cure the other sixty, more easily and securely, and in shorter time. His success was amazing. Look, also, at the practice of the German peasant, Priessnitz, which, however unnatural it may appear to those who have not investigated the subject, and to others who have all their lifetime outraged nature, by living in opposition to her laws, proves, by its stupendous effects, that it is built on the soundest and most rational physiological principles. Where, in the history of drugs and drug doctors, shall we find a man, who, like him, has had under his charge nearly 3000 patients within two years (fourteen of whom were doctors), most of whom had exhausted the resources of science and drugs, who can say with him, that during that time he has not lost more than two individuals? In these days utility is every thing. We care not a rush for theories—give us results. Compare the above facts with cases treated by drugs in our hospitals, etc. But this plan has several other advantages: it is not revolting to the sense of taste—can be self-administered—every where procured—and, if not abused, is within the reach of all classes of the community.

As a proof of the growing estimation in which it is held, we refer to the facts, that there are already from twenty to thirty establishments, in different parts of this kingdom, most of which are presided over by very eminent medical men, who have relinquished the lucrative practice of drugs, the capabilities of which they were well acquainted with, and have embraced hydropathy. Among these we mention, with respect, Drs. E. Johnson, Courtney, Lovell, King, Sir E. Scudamore, Hume, Whetherhead, Wilson, Gully, Weiss, etc., etc. Besides which, a number of persons have, and are still practicing it privately, in their own houses, with very great advantages. (See Appendix, S.)

But notwithstanding the mass of evidence which has been produced in favor of the superior value of water as a therapeutic, it is in this, as in most other cases, where the parties concerned are influenced by prejudice and interest, the mind will be warped; for as Locke says, "Who, even by the most cogent arguments, will be prevailed with to disrobe himself at once of all his old opinions and pretences to knowledge and learning, which, with hard study he hath all his time been laboring for, and turn himself out stark naked, in quest of new notions? All the arguments that can be used will be as little able to prevail, as the wind was with the traveler to part with his cloak, which he held only the faster. It is, therefore, too much to expect the regular practitioner, who has very naturally great prejudices* against so great an innovation on his accustomed mode of thinking and acting, to adopt our plan, unless he had not a good practice on the old plan. On the other hand, as a medical writer says, "A comfortable medical practice is a very pleasant, easy-going business, which may be easily described: a compliment or two—a promise—and a prescription—and last, though not least, a guinea." This is the reason assigned, by the same author, why so few medical men are found conducting the water cure, for he seems reluctant to ascribe it to their want of discernment, to discover its superiority over that of drugs. But even some of those who have adopted hydropathy, and who had long enjoyed the monopoly of drugging the people, are exceedingly annoyed at finding their "vested right" unceremoniously invaded by persons of the "lower orders of society—some from among tinkers, or tailors, or teetotal messengers, or any others who have nothing else to do." These *un*professional men who write upon and practice the water cure are severely reprimanded, as "acting from purely selfish motives." Whereas in scores of instances they have absolutely no remuneration whatever, except that arising from the alleviation of the sufferings of their fellow-men. Besides, charges of this kind come with a very bad grace from such men as Dr. Graham, etc., who have enriched themselves by their enormous charges for advice, etc., no more calculated to benefit the patient than that given by these *un*professional tinkers, etc., etc. "Physician, heal thyself" of selfishness, and refrain from throwing stones, till you have secured your own

* Dr. Bigel, of Strasburg, says, It must be remembered that I am a doctor, and that pride must suffer by receiving lessons from so humble a source as that of a peasant. And speaking of the conduct of medical men, in reference to hydropathy, he says, I shall not look for the motives, lest I should not find them of the most honorable nature; but will content myself with observing that its too great simplicity was, and still is, its only fault. The learned fear to be robbed of their science—the practitioner of his connection—and the apothecaries tremble for their shops and drugs.

windows. But what is implied in all this outcry against non-professional men, in which we are sorry to find some of our hydropaths are joining? Why, though it is indisputable that great good has resulted from the efforts of those persons on whom contempt is sought to be brought by calling them opprobious names, these results have not been produced by medical men. The monopoly has been broken in upon—their craft is in danger. It was not a doctor,* but a teetotal messenger, etc. Fudge! What is the difference to a sick man, whether it was a "tinker, tailor, teetotal messenger," etc., or a fellow of some learned university who was dubbed with an M.D., that found out, or employed, the means of making or keeping him well. We are advocates for an enlightened view of things. Truth fears nothing so much as concealment, and desires nothing so much as clearly to be laid open to the view of all. Truth will successfully assert its own supremacy—bear ultimately its proper sway on the subject; and demonstrate, to the satisfaction of all persons of discernment, and free from prejudice, that the system now considered is of great efficacy, and one worthy of the entire confidence of the public."† Let us not then withhold any thing on this subject, which we know to be true, though it may entail abuse, misrepresentation, and a variety of disagreeables which most men are naturally anxious to avoid. But there are too many who

* The practice of physic has been more improved by the casual experiment of illiterate nations, and the rash ones of vagabond quacks, than by the reasonings of all the once celebrated professors of it, and theoretic teachers in the several schools of Europe; very few of whom have furnished us with one new medicine, or have taught us better how to use our old ones, or have in any instance at all improved the art of curing diseases.—*Dr. Heberden's Medicine.*

Reform not often proceeds from within, and in no time or country did it ever make progress, unless assisted from without.—*Dr. Dickson.*

† Dr. Graham. This gentleman regards hydropathy only as an auxiliary to drugs. This, however, is in direct opposition to several very eminent and successful hydropaths, who are of opinion that mixing the water treatment with that of drugs, is highly dangerous; may cost the patient his life; and cannot fail to bring hydropathy into contempt.

feel like the French king, who said, "These matters, however bad, and however destined to be removed by man's enlightenment, will last my time, and serve my purpose. *Apres nous le Deluge.*" Is this right? Are we to hold our peace when evil is rampant, and choose ease rather than usefulness?—personal convenience rather than the public good? Away with such views! Spurn them with the contempt they deserve, and "work while it is called to-day." Expect, however, that you will meet with opposition; for though we are grieved that it should be so, yet so it is, that giving offence to some parties in making known any novelty, or seeking to introduce or extend any improvement, cannot be avoided. This is the natural consequence of things. "Persecution has ever been the reward of truth, before that truth has made itself fashionable."* "And whosoever shall move one step beyond the line of the world's convention, must expect to meet with the thundering anathemas and obloquies of all who wish to stand well with the arbiters of public opinion."† Persecution is the last resource of those, who, conscious that they cannot defend themselves and their practices by logic, employ brute force. And whenever you see a disputant in a rage, and hear him threaten, you may be sure he feels he is beaten in argument: hence, if he can, he turns persecutor, this being his forlorn hope. The ingenious De Foe says, "He that opposes his judgment against the consent of the times, ought to be backed with unanswerable truths; and he that hath truth on his side is a fool as well as a coward, if he be afraid to own it, because the currency of the multitude‡ of other men's opinions." "In proportion as

* Dr. F. Lees, the teetotal champion.

† Bentham.

‡ An error is not the better for being common, nor truth the worse for having lain neglected; and if it were put to the vote any where in the world, I doubt, as things are managed, whether truth would have the majority: at least while the authority of men, and not the examination of things must be its measure.—*Locke.* Truth has nothing to do with numbers, but with knowledge and correct judgment. Nothing is more clear from history, than that in most things the majority is in the wrong.

any branch of study leads to important and useful results—in proportion as it gains ground in public estimation—in proportion as it tends to overthrow prevailing errors—in the same degree it may be expected to call forth any declamation from those who are trying to despise what they will not learn, and wedded to prejudices which they cannot defend. Galileo probably would have escaped persecution, if his discoveries could have been disproved, and his reasonings refuted."

How often have we heard persons exclaiming when the doctor has sent his compliments, etc., at Christmas,

> "Oh! what a bill!
> Here's half-a-crown for draught and pill,
> Which did not cost him two pence."

And though the people have been more to blame in this matter than the doctor, they are now beginning to open their eyes to the value of cold water—they see

> "That's the best physic which doth cure our ills,
> Without the charge of 'pothecaries' bills."

There are, however, multitudes who still estimate and remunerate the service of their professional attendant by no other criterion than the quantity of drugs they have taken.*

* Of a great many anecdotes told us by one well acquainted with English medical practice, we shall select one as an illustration of the extent of prejudice existing upon this subject, and its effects in corrupting practitioners. An elderly lady received a hurt in her arm, which required the attendance of a medical practitioner, residing at two or three miles' distance. He dressed it about twenty times, and saw it completely healed. Now was his time to consider how he should be paid. My only chance, said he to himself, is to begin ordering medicine. He therefore affected to think unfavorably of the appearance of the skin of her arm: it betokened a bad state of the blood. I shall send you something for it, said he. He now began a course of medicine, to which the old lady very willingly submitted; at length it amounted to nine pounds; he admitted she was well, and sent in his bill. When he next called, she told him she had got the bill, and was wishing to pay it. "But I think," said she, "you must surely have committed a mistake in draw

Nay, they even boast of the quantity they have taken in a given time. How frequently do we hear the finish tint given to their credulity: "The doctor said if I had not had a constitution like a horse, I never could have stood it:" and he might have added: "Had you not the mind of an ass, you never would." But without being too sanguine, may we not hope to live to see the day when the good sense of the people will induce them to abandon those "innocent? deceptive medicines, which are in many cases given to please the patient"—that we shall hear wholesale druggists declare that "times are bad," that "water is *riz* and drugs are fell"—that young dentists, before they get old, will be surprised to find that there is not so much toothache—that whole sets are not destroyed at a sitting, by mercury and calomel; or by slower degrees, though with equal effect, by hot tea, coffee, etc.; and animal food, as in the days of yore—that drugs will be like the Latin language, a dead letter, or like some other things, be rendered obsolete by time and the progress of man's enlightenment—that the service of a vast majority of medical men will be dispensed with as useless, and the few who remain to direct the agency of cold water, shall enjoy the full confidence of an enlightened temperate people, and be cheerfully and liberally compensated in exchange for scientific truth, not for "murderous drugs."

That we are not singular, or so much so as some imagine, we refer to the declaration of a few, whose testimony may have some weight with the public. Dr. Orphen says, "Every

ing it out." "What seems wrong, madam?" inquired he. "If there be any error, of course we can easily rectify it!" "Oh, why, you have nine pounds here for medicine—that is all very well—I have had that. But you have three pounds ten for dressing my arm. Now you know, I had nothing there. You were only put to a little trouble, which was the same as nothing. I cannot understand this part of your bill at all!" "Oh! very well!" said he, "if you think so, we'll deduct the charge for dressing!" It is needless to add that the balance was ample remuneration for his service, as well as for his medicines!—*Chambers' Edinburgh Journal, No.* 34, *New Series.*

year adds to my conviction that if the public would act with common sense, and relinquish those drinking habits which have so long domineered over society, they would enjoy such a portion of health as would starve almost all the physicians. This is my simple statement," says he, "*contrary to my own personal interest and advantage.*" And Dr. Courtney says, "Plain, wholesome food, and the pure element, water, and nothing stronger, should ever enter the system, and take my word for it, whoever follows this system, will seldom want a doctor. The teetotalers [especially those of them who have taken the third stage] are the very worst customers the doctor ever had. They will close the shops of the doctors as fast as they will the breweries." The "Times," in reviewing Mr. Claridge's work on hydropathy, says, "Apothecaries Hall, our next door neighbor, to which we have often resorted for relief, and departed under a notion that we obtained it, now totters to a fall on the fiat of a Silesian peasant." The "Era" also observes; "If one tithe of the beneficial effects adduced by Mr. Claridge, from the simple element, cold water, can be substantiated, we can only say, let the doctors look to themselves, or they will ere long have a roughish time of it." Of hydropathy, therefore, we may say with great propriety and assurance:

"Great doctor! the art of curing 's cured by thee;
We now thy patient physic see
From all inveterate diseases free;
Purged of old errors by the cure,
New dieted, put forth to clearer air;
It now will strong and healthful prove;
Itself before lethargic lay, and could not move."—*Old Poem.*

As, however, those who are "advocates for an enlightened view of things," must, in carrying out their principles, in endeavoring to make converts to their opinions, necessarily have up-hill work for a time, and sometimes "break a lance for their opponents, yea, even receive a few scars in the bloodless encounter," we must console ourselves as well as we can, and "heal all their scratches with water."

PART IV.

CHAPTER IX.

AIR.

The enjoyment of free air may be considered as a nourishment equally necessary for our existence as eating and drinking. Pure air is essentially the greatest means of strengthening and supporting life; while confined and corrupted air is the most subtle and deadly poison.—DR. HUFELAND.

THERE are few circumstances essential to the preservation of health, to which so little attention is generally paid, as the breathing of pure air. A short explanation of the manner in which the atmosphere acts on the animal body, will probably be the best means of impressing on the mind of the reader the importance of a due supply of this first necessary of life. In doing this we shall be as brief as possible.

The air we breathe is a subtle and fluid substance, which surrounds every part of the globe, and which all living beings respire, either by the lungs, the pores of the skin, or by both.*

* Respiration, says Professor Liebig, is the falling weight, the bent spring which keeps the clock in motion; the inspirations or expirations are the stroke of the pendulum which regulate it. In our ordinary timepieces, we know, with mathematical accuracy, the effect produced on their rate of going, by changes in the length of the pendulum, or in the external temperature. Few, however, have a clear conception of the influence of air and temperature on the health of the human body; and yet the research into the conditions necessary to keep it in the normal state is not more difficult than in the case of a clock. Dr. E. Johnson says, Respiration is as certainly performed by the skin as the lungs, and that nothing can be more certain than that nature, in her anxiety to insure a

It is the element to which the animal and vegetable world owes its life, beauty, and preservation. All the changes which we see take place in different beings here below, depend upon air. It is so needful to the existence of animals, that the greater part of them could not live more than half a minute if they were deprived of it; and the others could not, generally, bear the want of it more than two days. It is necessary to the birds of the air, and the fish of the sea; and even plants, in order to vegetate, have need of air. Sounds could not be propagated without it, nor could winds be formed. The sun itself could not furnish us with either a sufficiency of light or heat, if the air did not surround our globe.

Every square inch of the surface of the globe is pressed by a column of air of fifteen pounds weight; every square foot, by one of 2160 pounds; and a middle-sized man, whose surface is about fourteen feet, carries a load of atmospheric air, equal to 30,240 pounds weight! By means of heat the air may be made to occupy a space of 550,000 times greater than that which it occupies in its common atmospheric state.

full and perfect accomplishment of the all-important functions of respiration, has provided us with a double set of respiratory apparatus, viz., the lungs and the skin. As a proof of this, he refers to experiments, which have shown that the animal breath consists of carbonic acid, the vapor of water, and nitrogen. And that the same experiments of the same experimenters, have proved that the exhalations from the body—the breath of the skin—is also composed of the same constituents—carbonic acid, vapor of water, and nitrogen—and that, therefore, perspiration and respiration, as the very words themselves would indicate, are essentially the same. Liebig also says, from the first moment that the functions of the lungs, or of the skin, are interrupted or disturbed, compounds, rich in carbon, appear in the urine—that carbon which ought to have been given off either by the lungs or by the skin, whichever of the two happen to be in fault. But important as the skin is, as our assistant organ of respiration, we utterly deprive ourselves of its assistance, by the absurd fashion of our dress, and the ridiculous care with which we defend the skin from all access of atmospheric air—thus, to a large extent, shutting out the oxygen so vitally essential to life; and shutting in the carbonic acid, which is known to be so deadly to all animal, and also to vegetable life. When shall we learn to be wise? "When shall it once be?"

This air is a compound of different airs, called gases; of which a gas called oxygen (and sometimes from its being indispensable to the maintenance of animal life, vital air) forms twenty-one parts in every 100; the remaining seventy-nine parts being a gas called nitrogen, or azote. The air which is drawn into the lungs in the act of breathing, and through the pores of the skin, acts on the blood, which is returned through the veins from different parts of the body, so as to change it from dark purple to a light scarlet. In this process the oxygen disappears, having formed chemical combinations with certain substances contained in the venous blood, by which it is changed partly into a gas, called carbonic acid gas, and partly into water. A minute proportion of this gas is consequently found in the present air we meet with. The carbonic acid gas is not only unfit for the support of life, but it is positively a poison, since a given proportion of the atmospheric air will support an animal much longer, if this gas be removed as fast as it is formed, than if it be suffered to remain. By the abstraction of the substance from which these new combinations are formed, the blood is purified and rendered fit to stimulate to proper action the nerves and muscles; to restore the structure of the various portions of the body, which are continually becoming useless, and being removed, to furnish the secretions, as they are called, by which the process of digestion, and other processes necessary to the existence of our bodies are performed. In short, to use the emphatic language of Scripture, which has been quoted and illustrated by the greatest physiologists of this country, "the blood is the life thereof;" and the blood itself loses its vitality, if it be not continually purified by exposure to the action of atmospheric air.

From the above it will be evident, that if an animal be confined to a given quantity of air, every time the act of breathing is repeated, that air is contaminated, and is becoming less fit for the proper performance of the process above described. Every time the blood circulates it consequently gets more impure, and less capable of stimulating the heart, and other organs, to action. The circulation becomes more languid, till the heart ceases to beat, and the animal dies. This truth might be proved by reference to such facts as—the short time during which a person can exist in a diving-bell—the well-known story of the black-hole, or, prison of Calcutta—and circumstances which have occurred and are still occurring in the accursed African slave trade.

It is calculated that every individual consumes about five cubic feet of air in an hour, or in other words, deprives such a quantity of air of its oxygen, or vital principle. If a hundred persons, therefore, were confined in a room thirty feet long, twenty-five broad, and thirty high, the whole of the air in that apartment, consisting of 22,500 cubic feet, unless renewed, would be rendered noxious in about four hours and a half. By an experiment of the celebrated Hales, a gallon of air was consumed, or spoiled, by the steam of the breath, in one minute, so as to be unfit for respiration; hence a hogshead, or sixty-three gallons, would hardly supply a human being for an hour.

There are several very interesting and ably written articles in that excellent periodical, the "Christian Witness," on this subject, which will amply repay the attention of the reader. The appeal is to the women of England, on behalf of 300,000 young men and boys, engaged in the various branches of trade and industry in the metropolis, and suffering by the late-hour system. Their condition is described with great minuteness, and shown to be painful in the extreme. Employed for sixteen, or seventeen, or more hours every day, in shops badly ventilated, nearly filled with customers for several hours, at night having twenty or thirty gas-burners, each consuming as much oxygen as four persons, always standing on their legs, compelled to take their three meals in half an hour—all this must, in the end, be ruinous to the health of those who are compelled to endure it. The air they breathe in the daytime is decidedly bad, and becomes gradually more and more impure, until in the evening, when the doors are closed, the shop more crowded, and the gas burning, it becomes positively and actively pernicious. The results of such a state of things may be easily inferred. The lungs imperfectly perform their functions; as a necessary consequence, the blood is only partially oxygenized, or changed from the venous into the arterial; the circulation becomes sluggish; all the secretions are rendered impure by the impurity of the blood; digestion is impaired; the muscular system is weakened; and the whole physical constitution becomes, in a greater or less degree, the subject of chronic disease. This subject is now, happily, exciting great interest, and we beseech our readers to peruse the articles above referred to for themselves. Let them do it without delay, and act upon their convictions.

Is it not also surprising, that while we take so much care about our food, we should not bestow even more attention upon an article equally, if not more, essential to health and enjoyment? Hence the absurdity of endeavoring to make our rooms air tight—of huddling ourselves up in a large quantity of clothes* by day and by night—and in the latter case, of surrounding ourselves with close-drawn bed curtains, as if we actually wanted to stifle ourselves. We do not act so foolishly with the delicate and fragile plants in our gardens. As it has been beautifully said, " See how they are buffeted by the wind,

* The case adverted to by Dr. E. Johnson is not of uncommon occurrence. He says—" I got into a coach a mile from London, the other day, because there was no room outside. The weather was dry, but cold and sharp. In the corner of the coach there sat a mighty combination of bone and muscle, thew and sinew, all assisting in the formation of what should have been a man. He was at least six feet high, and 'bearded like a pard;' and seemed as well able to carry the coach as the coach was to carry him! As soon as I entered the vehicle, I let down the window; but before I had succeeded in doing so, there issued, from amidst the cloaks, and coats, and shawls, and wrappings, and mufflings, in which this great thing had enveloped itself, a voice of supplication and woe: 'For God's sake do not let the window down! I am so susceptible—so extremely susceptible!' Had he been as capable of thinking as he was susceptible of feeling, he would have seen he was the author of the evil of which he complained."

and alternately scorched by the sun, and deluged by the rain, and frozen by the frost, and spattered by the mud, and brushed and bruised by the passenger's foot! Yet how greenly and healthily they grow! Take them into your parlor, and warm them by the fire, and curtain them with flannel,* and defend them from the cold, and the wind, and the rain, and the rude contact of the traveler's foot, and the other 'discomforts' of this out-of-door existence. What think you, will they continue to flourish as greenly and as healthily as before? 'Oh! but,' say you, 'there is a difference between a man and a cabbage!' A difference! why, I know there are many differences! A man does not bear leaves and look green; a cabbage has neither arms nor legs; and though it has as good a heart as many who rejoice in the name and nature of man, still that heart contains no blood. But what of all this? To constitute analogy, it is not necessary that there should be agreement in every particular. At this rate there would be no analogy between man and woman, nor even between man and man; for there are, probably, no two men in existence exactly alike. But, in all that concerns our present purpose, the man and the plant are perfectly analogous; they are both living beings, destined to exist under certain circumstances—living systems, destined to occupy a certain position within the circumference of that circle of existence which constitutes the universal whole. Those who are not conversant with animal and vegetable phys-

* Mr. Beamish, speaking of the action of the atmosphere on the surface of the skin, says: "There is not one of these surfaces which is not permeable to the external air, nor is there one of the elementary cells of our body which does not absorb and elaborate the atmospheric gases, thereby disengaging and absorbing caloric by turns. Hence the injurious effect of wearing flannel next the skin; for, by preventing the action of the atmosphere, it effectually stops the elaboration of caloric by that organ, weakens its tissues, and throws often an overpowering amount of labor upon the lungs, producing, first, functional derangement, and ultimately, organic changes. What would be said if a piece of flannel were constantly worn upon the mouth? And yet this would be about as philosophical as applying it to the skin.

iology, will be astonished, upon examination, to find how little, indeed, is the real and essential difference between plants and animals. In all, life is the same—more or less complex, but still the same; consisting, in all, of a number of effects, resulting from and depending upon the four grand conditions of matter: viz., organism, contractility, sensibility, and stimuli."

Dr. Bigel observes: "Air is the food of the lungs, being the same to them as food is to the stomach;" and Dr. Hufeland even goes so far as to assert, that there is a great accession of vital nourishment from without, which is received by our lungs and skin, and which is of much more importance than the nourishment received by the stomach.

The Abbe Sanctorius, a Florentine, who was well qualified to give an opinion, supports the same view. He was upward of twenty years engaged in determining what quantity of perspiration ought to pass from the body when in a healthy state. To ascertain this, he placed small glasses, some not larger than thimbles (having first cleaned and weighed them), on various parts of the body, when, after indefatigable research, the result proved that every man ought to pass from his body daily, from six to seven pounds; two pounds and a half are supposed to pass by the ordinary means of evacuation, and the remainder by the pores of the skin. (See Appendix, T.) But as few persons take more than one pound and a half of solids, and two pounds of liquids, into their stomachs in a day, the question now arises, whence this great residue originates? the answer is, that men, like all other organic things, feed upon air. If this be true, it follows, that much depends upon what sort of air we breathe; that of crowded or confined cities or rooms being productive of evil, while that of a fine open room and country contributes, as every one ought to know, to health, cheerfulness, and longevity.

Nothing is more common, and attended with more serious consequences, than common colds. They are generally produced by persons going from the external cold air into the warm air of a heated room, and not, as is generally supposed, by going out into the cold air. Hence we often hear persons express their fear of "taking cold," but never of "taking heat." When a person, in cold weather, goes into the open air, every time he draws in his breath the cold air passes through his nostrils and windpipe into the lungs, and consequently diminishes the heat of those parts. As long as he continues in the cold air he feels no bad effects from it; but as soon as he returns home he approaches the fire to warm himself, and very often takes some *Chinese soup*, or alcoholic drinks, to *keep the cold out*, as it is said. Now this is the very way to fix a cold in the head and chest, because of the sudden transition effected in the temperature of the parts by the incautious use of heat. The person soon feels a glow of heat within his nostrils and breath, as well as over the whole surface of the body, which is succeeded by a disagreeable dryness and huskiness felt in the nostrils and breast. By and by, a short, dry, tickling cough comes on; he feels a shivering, which induces him to draw nearer to the fire, but all to no purpose; for the more he tries to heat himself, the more he becomes chilled.

It should therefore be a rule with all persons, when they go into, or come out of, a very cold atmosphere, never to go directly from, or to, a room that has a fire in it; or if they cannot avoid that, to keep for a considerable time at the utmost distance from it; and above all, they should refrain, both before and after, from taking warm or strong liquors for some time.

The want of attention to pure air, has had a very prejudicial effect on the health of the community; hence it is computed, by qualified authorities, that the annual loss of life, from filth and bad air, is greater than the loss of life from death or wounds in any modern war in which this country has been engaged. The poor-law commissioners state, that of the 43,000 cases of widowhood, and of the 112,000 cases of destitute orphanage, relieved by the poor-rates of England and Wales alone, it appears that the greatest proportion of deaths of the heads of families occurred from removable causes—of which bad air forms one.

I have thus endeavored briefly to explain and enforce a very dark, complicated, and much-neglected subject, from the full conviction that there is no station in life in which some knowledge of it may not be of essential service, and that the practice to which the reader's attention has been directed would greatly tend to the preservation of health, and the attainment of longevity. And as the importance of the subject is very happily elucidated by the following anecdote, we shall conclude with it. It is said that the late Dr. Darwin, one day, at Nottingham, assembled a large crowd of people around him, and thus addressed himself to them: "Ye men of Nottingham! listen to me. You are ingenious and industrious mechanics. By your industry, life's comforts are procured for yourselves and families. If you lose your health, the power of being industrious will forsake you. That you know; but you do not know that to breathe fresh and changed air constantly, is not less necessary to preserve health than sobriety itself. Air becomes unwholesome in a few hours, if the windows are shut. Open those of your sleeping rooms whenever you quit them to go to your workshops. Keep the windows of your workshops open whenever the weather is not insupportably cold. I have no interest in giving you this advice. Remember what I, your countryman, and a physician, tell you. If you would not bring infection and disease upon yourselves, and to your wives and little ones, change the air you breathe; change it many times a day, by opening your windows."*

* In cases where persons cannot leave their room for more than a few minutes, the air may be changed, most effectually, by what is called pumping the room, which is done in the following manner: the doors and windows are put wide open, when a person, holding the door in his hand, violently swings it backward and forward. Thus, in a very short time, the bad air is exchanged for that which is fresh and pure. This may be done also in the cottages of the poor, even where their windows will not open, and where they have only one door.

PART V.

CHAPTER X.

EXERCISE.

The studious, the contemplative, the valetudinary, and those of weak nerves, if they aim at health and long life, must make exercise in a good air a part of their religion.—DR. CHEYNE.

I do not allow the state of the weather to be urged against the prosecution of measures so essential to health, since it is in the power of every one to protect themselves from cold by clothing, and the exercise may be taken in a chamber, with the windows thrown open, by actively walking backward and forward, as sailors do on shipboard. —ABERNETHY.

The wise, for cure, on exercise depend;
God never made his work for man to mend.—DRYDEN.

REVELATION, nature, reason, and high medical authority, all show the importance, and enforce the necessity of exercise. Hence we find the sovereign Father of the universe himself, his son Jesus Christ, and the eternal Spirit, engaged in a variety of works of providence and of grace. If from the Deity we descend to angels, they are described as the most active ministers of God, which "do his pleasure." And of the "great multitude" of redeemed souls, who come out of "great tribulation," we are told that they "rest not day and night," praising God.

Descending from heaven to earth, the same law seems impressed upon all. Our own nature, which owes its growth, its improvement, its health, and pleasures—nay, even society itself owes to exercise its being, its continuance, and its comforts. Yet not these alone enjoin the duty; for we are sent, by high authority, to the animal world, to read there, in the plainest language, the reproof of those who disregard the dictates of their own nature—who hide their hands in their bosoms, and refuse to labor. For the condemnation of such, Providence hath created one animal (the American sloth), the very opprobrium of the race, to hold up to scorn a vice which brings with it disease and misery, and "shall clothe a man with rags."

From the divine, the angelic, the rational, the animal nature, we might proceed to the inanimate world. The heavenly bodies, which are ever moving, and the elements composing this lower world, are all in the same useful motion, fulfilling the will of their great Creator, and bearing testimony against man's indolence. A wise and benevolent Author must possess some end in the production of his works; but this end, whatever it was, could never be promoted by inactivity, which is, in fact, the next in degree to non-existence. Even innocent Adam was put "into the garden of Eden to dress it, and to keep it," showing that, though we may have abundance of this world's good, we are not exempt from labor. Motion is the soul of the universe, which is governed by the same laws as man. Hence, that the air and sea may not become injurious to the earth and its inhabitants, by the corruption which a dead stillness would produce, they are violently agitated, not by the gentle, light winds, but by storms and tempests, which purify the whole. Thus—

"By ceaseless action, all that is subsists;
Constant rotation of the unwearied wheel
That nature rides upon, maintains her health,
Her beauty, her fertility. She dreads an instant's pause,
And lives but while she moves."

Cowper's Task.

The structure of man's body,* as well as of his mind, plainly

* Addison, after giving a description of the human body, says, "The general idea of an animal body, without considering it in its niceties of anatomy, let us see how absolutely necessary exercise is for the right preservation of it. There must be frequent motions and agitations, to mix, digest, and separate the juices contained in it, as well as to clear

shows that he was never intended for a merely contemplative life; and a thousand instances prove that exercise, health, and longevity are inseparable. Those whom poverty obliges to labor for daily bread are not only the most healthy, but generally the most happy, and the longest livers. Industry and sobriety seldom fail to place them above want, and water, air, and exercise, the three best doctors, serve them instead of physic. This is more peculiarly the case with those who live by the culture of the ground, and are consequently much exposed to all sorts of weather, and who take much exercise.

The love of activity shows itself very early in man. So strong is this principle, that the healthy youth cannot be restrained from it, even by the fear of punishment; and this love of motion is surely a strong proof of its utility, because nature implants no dispositions in vain. It seems to be a universal law, through the whole animal creation, that no being, without exercise, should enjoy health, or be able to find subsistence. Every creature, except man, takes as much of it as is necessary. He alone, and such animals as are under his control, deviate from this original law, and hence suffer the just consequences.

Inactivity never fails to induce a universal relaxation of the solids, which disposes the body to innumerable diseases; for when the solids are relaxed, neither digestion nor any of the secretions can be duly performed, in which case the worst consequences ensue. And how can persons, who loll about all day in easy chairs, and sleep long nights on beds of down, fail to be relaxed? Nor do such greatly mend the matter, who never stir abroad but in a coach, sedan, or such like. These elegant pieces of luxury are become so common, that the in-

and cleanse the infinitude of pipes and strainers of which it is composed, and to give their solid parts a more firm and lasting tone."

The number of muscles in the human body is 474, and that of the bones 247; and it is reasonable to conclude, that a very considerable degree of active corporeal exertion must be daily necessary, in order to afford sufficient exercise for so large a number of bodies, possessing great solidity, and expressly formed for action.

habitants of great towns seem to be in some danger of losing the use of their limbs altogether. It is now thought, by some, to be below any one to walk, who can afford to be carried. How ridiculous would it seem, to a person not acquainted with modern luxury, to behold the young and healthy swinging along on the shoulders of their fellow-creatures! or to see a fat carcass, overrun with disease occasioned by indolence and intemperance, dragged through the streets by half a dozen horses! And though many of them have not exercise enough to keep their humors wholesome, yet they dare not make a visit to their next-door neighbor but in a coach, or sedan, lest they should be looked down upon. Strange that men should be such fools as to be laughed out of the use of their limbs, and to throw away their health, in order to gratify a piece of vanity, or to comply with a ridiculous and injurious fashion! But we abound in absurdity and inconsistency: thus, though it is generally admitted that air and exercise are good, yet what means are made use of to avoid them! what stopping of crevices; what wrapping up in warm clothing; what shutting of doors and windows! Many London families go out once a day to take an airing, three or four in a carriage, one perhaps sick; they go five or six miles, or as many turns in Hyde Park, with the glasses both up, all breathing over and over again the same air they brought out of town with them in the carriage, with the least possible change, and rendered worse and worse every moment; and this they call taking exercise, or an airing! Our forefathers acted more wisely, and enjoyed the benefits arising therefrom.

> By chase our long-lived fathers earned their food,
> Toil strung their nerves, and purified their blood;
> But we, their sons, a pamper'd race of men,
> Are dwindled down to three-score years and ten.
> Better to hunt in fields, for health unbought,
> Than fee the doctor for a nauseous draught.—*Dryden.*

Voltaire gives us a very pleasant story of Caul, a voluptuary who could be managed with difficulty by his physician, and who, on finding himself very ill from indolence and intemperance, requested advice: "Eat a basilisk stewed in rose-water," replied the physician. In vain did the slaves search for a basilisk, until they met with Zadig, who, approaching Ogul, exclaimed, "Behold that which thou desirest; but my lord," continued he, "it is not to be eaten; all its virtues must enter through the pores. I have, therefore, inclosed it in a little ball, blown up, and covered with a fine skin; thou must strike this ball with all thy might, and I must strike it back again, for a considerable time, and by observing this regimen, and taking no other drink than rose-water, for a few days, thou wilt see and acknowledge the effect of my art." The first day Ogul was out of breath, and thought that he should have died of fatigue; the second he was less fatigued, and slept better; in eight days he recovered all his strength. Zadig then said to him, "There is no such thing in nature as a basilisk! but *thou hast taken exercise and been temperate, and hast therefore recovered thy health.*"*

Whosoever examines the accounts handed down to us of the greatest men, and of the longest livers, will generally find they were most exposed, lived on plain, coarse food, and took much exercise. This is often mentioned as something surprising in them, whereas the truth is, this is the cause of that which we wondered at, and had they accomplished what they did, under other circumstances, we might have wondered at it. Labor is neither disadvantageous or disgraceful, but profitable and honorable. The patriarchs and the distinguished sons of Jesse were shepherds, as were Moses and some of the prophets. Paul, though no mean scholar, was a tent maker. Cleanthes was a gardener's laborer, and used to draw water and spread it on his garden in the night, that he might have time to study during the day. He was the successor of Zeno. Æsop and Terence, whose names will live while lan-

* The remarks made by Sir C. Scarborough to the Duchess of Portsmouth, would apply to the bon vivant generally: "You must eat less—take more exercise—take physic—or be sick."

guage lives, were slaves. Cæsar studied in the camp, swam rivers, holding his writings out of the waters in one hand; while his clothing was spun and woven by his sisters. Mahomet made his own fires, swept his own house, milked his ewes, and mended his own shoes and pantaloons. Charlemagne, great in war, and greater in peace, filled his palace with learned men, founded schools and academies through his dominions, and yet was so industrious that he could frame laws even to the selling of eggs. Of Gustavus Vasa it is said, "A better laborer never struck steel."* Besides which we might refer to Alfred the Great, Dr. Franklin, Lord Monboddo, Louis Philippe,† the late king of the French, etc., etc. It is very doubtful if these men would ever have been so distinguished as they are, had they not been brought to the endurance of such privations and fatigues of body. These rendered their minds vigorous, their understanding clear, their perceptions acute, and all their mental faculties not only bright and elevated, but preserved them even in advanced life.

The immense advantage of exercise may be seen, if we consider that, "the more exercise any person takes, the larger is the quantity of oxygen he inhales, and the warmer he becomes; consequently the person who takes but little exercise, inhales but little oxygen, loses, in a great measure, its warming, vivifying, and strengthening agency. (See Appendix, U.) When there is a deficiency of oxygen in the system, the black

* It is astonishing what can be done by diligence and perseverance. The very earth trembles at the stroke of an undivided mind. That famous disturber and scourge of mankind, Charles XII. of Sweden, used to say, that, by resolution and perseverance a man might do every thing. Certainly he may do much more than at first setting out he thought it possible.

† Louis Philippe had been taught from his youth to wait upon himself; to despise all sorts of effeminacy; to sleep habitually on a wooden bed, with no covering but a mat; to expose himself to heat, cold, and rain; to accustom himself to fatigue by daily exercise, and by walking ten or fifteen miles with leaden soles to his shoes. See "Chambers' Miscellany of Useful and Entertaining Tracts."

blood from the veins is but imperfectly changed by the air in the lungs, and a blood unfit for the purposes of life flows through the body; the consequence of which is—must be—a falling off in the health to a greater or less extent. Hence arises those very prevalent affections—chilliness, languor, low spirits, headaches of different kinds, faintings, palpitations, stupor, apoplexy, etc."

In fact, so important and necessary is exercise, that without it, none of the various processes connected with the important functions of digestion could be properly performed. The health of all parts, and the soundness of their structure, depend on perpetual renovation; and exercise, by promoting at once absorption and secretion, invigorates life, renovates all the parts and organs, and renders them fit for all the purposes of health and longevity. It also mainly contributes to the proper circulation of the blood, and insures its imbibing the wholesome influences of the atmosphere, which, as shown above, form a principal source of our well-being. A brisk circulation animates the whole man, whereas deficient exercise, or continued rest, weakens the circulation, relaxes the muscles, diminishes the vital heat, checks perspirations, injures the digestion, sickens the whole frame, and thereby renders the individual subject to all attacks which disease may make upon him.

Indolence* not only occasions disease, and renders men useless to society, but actually injurious, for

> "Satan finds some mischief still,
> For idle hands to do.†"—*Watts.*

To say a man is idle is but little better than to say he is wicked. The mind, if not engaged in some useful pursuit, is

* Addison says, "An idle body is a monster in the creation; all nature is busy about him." A modern poet has beautifully shown that

> "Nature lives by toil;
> Beasts, birds, air, fire, the heavens and rolling worlds,
> All live by action: nothing lies at rest,
> But death and ruin. Man is born to care;
> Fashion'd, improved by labor."

There are but very few who know how to be idle and innocent.

constantly in quest of idle pleasure, or impressed with the apprehension of some imaginary evil. From these sources proceed most of the miseries of mankind. This applies particularly to the aged, who by no means ought to give way to a remission of exercise, since motion is the tenure of life. By degrees, the demand may sink to little more than a bare quit-rent; but that quit-rent must be paid, since life is held by the tenure.

The following reasons, in addition to what has been said before, show the value of exercise:

1. Your life will probably be prolonged by it. It is little less than suicide to neglect that, without doing which you are almost sure to shorten your days. The Creator has not so formed the body, that it can endure to be confined, without exercise, while the mind burns and wears upon its energies and powers every moment.

2. You will enjoy more with than without exercise. This remark is to be applied only to those who exercise daily; and to such it does apply with great force. Every one who is in this habit will bear ample testimony to this point.

3. You will add to the enjoyment of others. A cheerful companion is a treasure; and all will gather around you as such, if you are faithful to yourself; for exercise will make you cheerful, and cheerfulness will make you friends.

4. Your mind will be strengthened by exercise. The medical poet has justly observed,

> " 'Tis the great art of life to manage well
> The restless mind;"

and that by neglecting exercise, and injuring the bodily health, you also

> "The most important health,
> That of the mind, destroy."

Were you wishing to cultivate a morbid, sickly taste, which will, now and then, breathe out some beautiful poetic images, or thought, like the spirit of some most refined essence, too delicate to be handled or used in this matter-of-fact world, and too ethereal to be enjoyed, except by those of like palate, you shut yourself up in your room for a few years, till your nerves only continue to act, and the world floats before you as a dream. But if you wish for a mind that can fearlessly dive into what is deep, soar to what is high, grasp and hold what is strong, and move and act among minds conscious of its strength, firm in its resolve, manly in its aims and purposes, *be sure to be regular in taking exercise.*

We shall conclude our remarks on this head by a few of Dr. E. Johnson's concluding observations, in that invaluable work, "Life, Health, and Disease."

If you would preserve your health, therefore, exercise, severe exercise—proportioned, however, to your strength—is the only means which can avail you. Recollect, the body must be disorganized, wasted, sweated, before it can be nourished. With plentiful bodily exertion, you can scarcely be ill; without bodily exertion you cannot possibly be well. By "well," I mean the enjoying as much strength as your system is capable of—but by exertion and exercise, I do not mean the petty affair of a three miles' walk: I mean what I say—bodily exertion, to the extent of quickened breathing and sensible perspiration, kept up for three or four hours out of the twenty-four—say, four or five miles before breakfast, four or five before dinner, four or five early in the evening; or to save the evening for other purposes, a healthy man may walk a dozen miles before breakfast, with an advantage to himself which will, in a week or two, perfectly astonish him. Most men, even the operative manufacturers and shop keepers, may do this, if they will take the trouble to rise early enough; and fortunately the exercise taken before breakfast is worth all that can be taken afterward. (See Appendix, V.)

But—I beg your pardon—I must make another short quotation, which has this moment occurred to me—one which, though exceedingly short, embodies in itself the truth and wisdom of a hundred volumes: it is the following brief aphorism of the late Mr. Abernethy, with which I shall conclude—"If you would be well, live upon sixpence a day and earn it."

PART VI.

CHAPTER XI.

WATER AS A THERAPEUTIC, OR CURATIVE, AND THE VARIOUS MODES OF APPLYING IT.

Most blessed water! neither tongue can tell
  The blessedness thereof, no heart can think,
Save only those to whom it hath been given,
  To taste of that divinest gift of Heaven.
I stooped and drank of that divinest well,
  Fresh from the rock of ages where it ran;
It had a heavenly quality to quell
  All pain: I rose a renovated man;
And would not now, when that relief was known,
For worlds that needful suffering have forgone.

SOUTHEY.

NOTWITHSTANDING the efficacy of the hydropathic mode of treating diseases, if we consider the contempt in which every thing else is held, which is thought to be new, is it not surprising that many should be found skeptical as to its ultimate success? But amidst all the opposition with which it has had to contend, it has effected wonders, and produced an unparalleled sensation throughout the land.

Without attempting a defence of the water cure, which has been ably done by Drs. E. Johnson, Courtney, Wilson, etc., we shall pass on to give what appears to have been the most simple and efficacious plans pursued; reminding our readers, that those who are not suffering from hereditary disease, and who follow nature, will not need to have recourse even to these. In cases of diseases of long standing, of a complicated nature, and which affect the more vital parts of the body, it is not recommended to the patient to treat himself, but to place himself, if possible, under the care of some one who has studied, and understands the principles of the care.* We refer all those who wish to understand it, to the authors before named, by whom the principles are explained; the various modes of application given; and the practice defended; though not in that simple and plain manner we could have desired. This, however, may be accounted for, seeing they wrote for the information and direction of medical men, in whose hands they wish to keep the cure; hence the free use of medical technicality, with which their works abound.

Patients who perspire in the morning, should commence drinking small doses, at short intervals, during the process of sweating, in order to keep up and promote the perspiration, and to cool important internal organs. Too much should not be taken, as it would check perspiration. A short time after breakfast, one glass of cold water should be taken every quarter or half hour, according to circumstances. A copious use of cold water during meals, if you are resolved to use hot, fat, and indigestible food, cannot be too strongly recommended. Let each, however, test by experiment how much he ought to use, as he alone is judge in the case. One grand criterion by which he may judge of the proper quantity of water to be taken generally is, when shivering takes place—in which case the patient should cease for a time, and have recourse to exercise, the sure means of removing any ill effects.

Under the head of the internal uses of cold water, we may classify injections into the different parts of the body; such as the throat, ears, etc. The syringe† is of great importance in

* Though all curable diseases are curable by hydropathy, yet there are diseases, such as where the general system is so far weakened as not to have sufficient energy left to enable the patient to undergo the treatment—disease of the lungs—organic defects—where the patient can only be relieved.

† A bone syringe can be procured for ninepence, and used without a second person.

all diseases of the abdomen. In some dangerous cases, ten or twelve injections have been given in one day; but they should be used as sparingly as possible. They should seldom exceed one or two daily, and in some cases tepid water will answer better than cold, especially in commencing the treatment with very irritable persons.

The different processes of the cold water treatment consist in ablutions—the rubbing wet sheets—the wet sheet to lie in—wet bandages—sweating in the blankets—and the various baths. To promote and increase the effects of cold water, used internally, it is applied externally in a variety of ways, according to the objects to be fulfilled in the treatment. We may first mention the

GENERAL ABLUTIONS,

which should be used by all persons, in health to preserve it, and in disease to cure it. The best time for these is the morning, immediately after rising from bed, before dressing, and before the body has become chilled. The patient must take exercise afterward, if possible, in the open air. Very great invalids only may be allowed, after washing, to retire to bed. The time required is only about five minutes, and the method is very simple, and can do no harm. The mode of taking the ablution is as follows: The patient stands in a spacious vessel (so that the water which runs off may not soil the room—where this is of moment, a large thick cloth should be spread under the vessel, and extend some distance beyond it); the naked hand, or a large sponge, is dipped in the water, and conveyed briskly for some three or four minutes, over the whole surface of the body—the quicker the better. (See Appendix, W.) Water may also be poured on the head; but all persons, especially at first, are not able to bear the latter application.

Another plan is, the patient has a wet sheet (not well wrung out as for sweating), thrown over the head and body, which creates a sensation, or slight shock, and is an excellent tonic. In this he remains one, two, or three minutes, or even more, if there be much heat in the system; one or two persons should assist the patient in well rubbing the body while in the sheet, and also with a dry one after the wet one is removed. The rubbing should be applied more vigorously to the parts diseased, if any. If this course be regularly attended to, with drinking freely of cold water, it will be found of great value to persons suffering from gout, in its infancy, nervous irritability, or weakness of the skin, etc. Let any person try it, and he will soon become a convert to our opinions.

If there were arguments needed to convince any of its importance, to all classes of the community, we need only call attention to the structure of that most important, but grossly neglected organ—the skin. The importance of a correct performance of its functions, is thus clearly shown by Dr. E. Johnson. "When the great extent of the skin is considered—its structure—its great sensibility—its exceeding vascularity—and the great abundance of nerves with which it is supplied—it cannot be doubted, I think, that so elaborate a piece of machinery was constructed in order to fulfill some very important functions in animal life. And whatever those functions may be, it must manifestly contribute to the due performance of those functions to keep the skin clean, and have it frequently refreshed by general ablutions. And again, whatever its functions may be, it must, I think, materially interfere with them to have the skin constantly covered from contact with cold air, which all experience proves to be so invigorating to the system generally, and to have it perpetually smeared and choked up with the grease of perspiration. Thus the skin is seen to be the most important and extensive organ of the human body; the greatest medium for purifying it; and every moment a multitude of useless, corrupted, and worn-out particles evaporate through its numberless small vessels,* in an insensible

* Obstructed perspiration is the cause of many of the most painful disorders of mankind; which we shall be convinced of, if we consider that

manner. This secretion is inseparately connected with life, and the due circulation of the blood.

If we were in a state of nature, the outward air, by playing upon the surface of the skin, would dry up, and carry off this moisture, as soon as it reached that surface. But in our artificial state, the air never being permitted to blow upon our bodies, they being covered three or four deep, with wrappings of various sorts, to exclude that air, which we appear to dread as if it would be death, our skins become clogged, and, by degrees, as we get older, the accumulation of stucco increases, becoming daily more and more impervious, until at length we get crusted over with a substance similar to Roman cement, or plaster of Paris! And yet we expect to have our health! Impossible! Disease must be the consequence, sooner or later. On the other hand, were the state of the skin well attended to, these horrid complaints, the gout, rheumatism, nervousness, and a thousand other miseries, to which we are now subject, would cease to be; and the annoying visitation of colds would no longer afflict us. Ancient history tells us that the perspi-

a healthy person of middle station, perspires, within twenty-four hours, no less than from three to six pounds, as was proved by the experiments of Sanctorius, who, to ascertain this fact, passed more than twenty years of his life in the weighing chair. It is thus, that the system expels, through the pores, "noxious matters, which, if retained in the body by a constricted skin, cannot be otherwise than productive of serious consequences; for this extensive outside covering is a necessary outlet for the wastes of nature, and discharges, when in a healthy state, more than the lungs, bladder, and bowels together. By microscopic inspection, it is fully proved, that the surface of the skin resembles a very scaly fish; those scales are so small, that a space occupied by a grain of sand, will cover 250 of them. On examining one of these scales by a highly magnifying power, it is clearly seen that one scale covers 500 pores, or holes through which perspiration escapes; consequently, the space occupied by a grain of sand, say the twentieth part of an inch, includes and covers 125,000 pores. What then must the surface of the whole skin cover? This is beyond all calculation, equally true and wonderful. Hence, it is proved to a demonstration, that the skin is constructed to answer the most important purposes in the animal economy. See Dr. Graham "On the Skin."

ration from the body of Alexander the Great was sweet to the smell—something like as if it were perfumed. (See Appendix, X.) So are the exudations from the bodies of all persons in a perfectly clean and healthy state. They know no more what the word dyspepsia means, experimentally, than do their ploughboys: their days are unclouded, their nights undisturbed, and existence to them is real delight. On the other hand, the skin being the seat of feeling, persons whose skin is weak have generally a sensation much too delicate for either health or enjoyment; they laugh or cry at the veriest trifles, showing great mental as well as physical weakness; and are so internally and externally afflicted by every variation of the atmosphere, that at length they become real barometers. Such a constitution is called the rheumatic, and arises chiefly from want of strength in the skin to perform its functions. It is also not to be forgotten, that the skin is the grand assistant of nature, in the removal, as well as in the prevention of disease; and that a man with open pores, and a skin sufficiently vigorous, may depend on being cured much more easily, and with more certainty. Without a sound skin, there can be no complete restoration.

That such an organ must be a great support of health and longevity, no one can deny; and it is therefore astonishing that, with all our progress in knowledge, we should have neglected it so much; that, instead of paying that attention to it which its importance demands, we should, from our infancy, have done every thing in our power to relax and weaken it, and to stop up its pores. Hence we have neglected washing and rubbing all over us, bathing, etc., and have substituted warm rooms, beds, and clothing. Is not this irrational? and when we pursue quite a different course with our horses, is it not unaccountable? The most ignorant person is convinced that proper care of the skin is indispensably necessary for the existence and well-being of horses, and of various other animals. The groom often denies himself sleep, and other gratifications, that he may curry his horses sufficiently. If they become meagre and weak, the first reflection is, whether there may not have been some neglect in regard to cleaning them. Such a simple idea, however, never occurs to him in respect to his children. If they grow feeble and sickly, if they pine away and are afflicted with worms in the external parts of the body, all the consequence of dirtiness,* he thinks rather of drugs, of witchcraft, and of other absurdities, than of the real cause—that is, neglecting to keep the skin clean and hard, by washing, rubbing, and exposure to the air as much as possible. Since we show so much prudence and intelligence in regard to animals, why not in regard to man?

Ablutions, though alone of great value, in some cases, are for the most part preparations for a more powerful system of treatment. The first five or six may be tepid; afterward they should be quite cold. Continued for a quarter of an hour, or longer, they act as a stimulant and refrigerant; if for a shorter time, they have a strengthening and exhilarating effect, and tend to equalize the circulation of the blood. They are fitted for all constitutions, even for women, children, and persons of old age. After ablutions, as regards mildness of operations, follow the various baths; as the

ORAL BATH,

which consists in regularly rinsing the mouth with water, which is retained for several seconds, and, by bending the head backward, is brought in contact with the posterior faucus, which also requires cleansing. This bath deserves especial recommendation, as an excellent tonic, a purifier of the mucous mem-

* "We speak from experience," says Dr. M. Syder, "when we declare it to be our opinion, that if both sexes were to wash their whole bodies as often as they do their hands and faces, they would escape a multitude of diseases, local as well as general, or constitutional. Inferior animals set us an example in this respect; yet 'reasoning man' is a more filthy animal than can be found in the creation. If we pursue him in his whole length of life, a pig (filthy as it is) is a clean, delicate piece of animation to him."

brane and salivary glands; its salutary effects extend, also, to the remote organs, which are not brought in contact with the water. The

NASAL BATH

consists in repeatedly drawing cold water up the nose, and again expelling it; and is of great use in colds of the head, in solving obstructions, and strengthening the structures.

SHOWER BATHS

are generally understood, if not sufficiently used. Very weak persons had better begin their use with tepid water, and they will soon prefer cold. They are of great use in diseases requiring repeated sweatings for their cure, and for patients who, in consequence of congestions, and diseases of the chest, cannot bear the full baths after the process of sweating. They should be in common daily use in all families, who wish to keep out of the hands of the doctor.

THE RUBBING WET SHEET

is of essential service. The sheet, when used in rubbing, is not so well wrung out as when otherwise used. The patient standing, it is thrown over the head and body, which creates a slight shock; friction is then used actively, by the patient (if able), and by an attendant. (See Appendix, Y.) This is continued for one or five minutes. After the sheet is removed, the process is completed by friction with a dry sheet, till a glow is produced. This is a fine tonic, and has been very useful to Sir F. B—n and others, who, though induced reluctantly to try it, were perfectly astonished at its effects.

THE WET SHEET TO LIE IN

is one of the principal means employed in the hydriatic treatment. A large, coarse linen sheet is dipped in cold water, well wrung out, and spread smoothly upon a mattrass upon which a blanket has been previously laid; the patient reclines upon this sheet, and the body is then carefully enveloped in it. It should be wound tight round the body. Two or three blankets should then be thrown over the patient, and well tucked in, so as to exclude the air. (See Appendix, Z.) If this does not sufficiently promote perspiration, let a light feather-bed be added. The first impression of the sheet is certainly disagreeable; the feeling of cold, however, passes away in about a quarter of a minute, or rather more, in cases where the patient has not much animal heat, and is then succeeded by a pleasant coolness, a genial warmth, and ends in perspiration. This, however, is not at all times desirable. The nature of the disease, and the object to be gained, must determine this case, as also the time the patient should remain in the covering.

The wet sheets are of remarkable utility in all febrile diseases. In acute fevers they must be changed according to the degree of heat—perhaps every quarter of an hour—until the dry, hot skin of the patient becomes softer, and more prone to perspiration. When that symptom is observed, the renewal of the wet sheet may be delayed for a longer period, until perspiration actually ensues. The patient must then remain for several hours in this state, until uneasy sensations and other inconveniences render it necessary to extricate him; but it is more advisable to keep him in the loosened envelopment until perspiration ceases spontaneously, when a tepid ablution, or half bath, should follow. This mode of treatment immediately abstracts morbid heat, lowers the pulse, relieves headache, and thirst in most cases, and that without in any degree enfeebling any function of the frame. If there should be headache, let it be removed by cold applications to the part; or if the feet remain cold for a long time, let them be wrapped in a dry blanket. In acute eruptions of the skin—measles, scarletina, small-pox, etc.—the wet sheets are not less serviceable, when the eruption cannot make its way to the surface, in consequence of the dry state and heat of the skin, and of the violence of the fever, or where the rash has receded suddenly, owing to other disturbances. In both cases the wet sheets are of essential service; one application of them suffices sometimes to re-establish the eruption. If the rash fail to make its appearance after the first or second envelopment, cold affusion is to be preferred. In a hot summer's day, after a long, but not very fatiguing walk, few things can exceed the refreshing, calming influence of a wet sheet. It is then far more refreshing than a tepid bath. It instantly cools the surface, relieves the spirits, and induces sleep; these effects render it of eminent service in nervous affections, and some states of diseased minds.

SWEATING IN THE BLANKET

is another mode of producing perspiration, and is perhaps the most disagreeable part of the treatment; although the patient soon becomes reconciled to it, because the unpleasant sensations are succeeded by the relief occasioned by the commencement of perspiration, which is much increased by the air that enters by the window, which at this time may with impunity be thrown open. (See Appendix, AA.) The mode is, the patient is enveloped in a large coarse blanket, the legs extended, and the arms kept close to the body; the blanket is then wound round it as tight as possible, confining it well at the neck and under the feet, that the heat given off by the body may be well retained. Over this is placed, and well tucked in, another blanket or two, and then a small feather-bed; finally a counterpane is spread over all, to promote perspiration. As soon as this appears, the windows are thrown open, and the patient allowed a wine-glass of cold water every half hour. Diseased parts are bandaged with a damp cloth before the patient is enveloped in the sheet. If headache be induced, a damp cloth is applied. The duration of the sweating depends on the nature of the disease and the constitution of the individual. In most cases, the patient has sweated long enough when the perspiration breaks out on the face; when the attendant takes off all but the blanket, in which the patient proceeds to the bath in straw shoes, having the face, and those parts of the legs and feet which are exposed to the air, damped with a cold wet cloth. Having arrived there, he washes his head, neck, and chest, and then plunges into the bath, where he remains from two to six minutes. Some people sweat every day, others alternate days, or only on the third day. The redness induced in the spine of the patient, after using the cold bath, is considered the touchstone to determine the strength the patient possesses to contend with the disease. Many patients are not allowed to sweat at all—perhaps not more than one half—and considerable difference as to the time is observed. Some are kept in the blankets for an hour—two hours—and some even three. Some will perspire in a quarter of an hour, while others require from three to five hours for that purpose. This treatment is of great service in gout, rheumatism, fever, scrofula, cutaneous diseases, and many other complaints. The morning, from four to six o'clock, is the best time for sweating. After the bath, patients who can walk, or take other exercise, should dress quickly, go into the open air, drink cold water, and afterward take a rational breakfast.

THE HALF BATH

is generally used as a stimulant and tonic, when the full bath would be too powerful for the patient—and serves as a preparative to it. (See Appendix, BB.) The water is between fifty-nine and seventy-seven degrees of Fahrenheit; from three to six inches deep; continued from five minutes to an hour; and generally employed after the patient has been in the wet sheet. He sits down in it, and cold water is either sprinkled or poured over him, after which, friction, and exercise in the open air, must be actively used. If this bath be intended as a preparation for more active treatment, it must be of short duration; but if the object be to produce a derivative effect—to remove congestions from other organs—the duration of the baths must be regulated by the effects. The patient must remain in them until revulsion is produced.

THE FULL BATH

is sometimes used after the sweating process, at other times without the previous part of the treatment. The effects are stimulating and strengthening, but it also acts as a powerful depressor; it is necessary, therefore, that sufficient vital energy should exist in the patient using it, to produce a full and proper degree of reaction after its employment. It also requires caution, and should never be taken, if there is reason to doubt the capabilities of the person being able to withstand the sudden depressing effects, or where there is congestions, inflammations of the internal organs, or diseases of the chest. The patient, after wetting his head and chest quickly, should enter the bath at once, as "delay is dangerous." Half a minute, or one minute, is generally sufficient.

THE PLUNGING BATH

may be taken, by the patient who is not able to plunge himself, by being laid upon a sheet held by several persons, which is quickly plunged into the water, and again withdrawn. The object of these baths is nearly the same as that of the former, but their action is more stimulating. One, or, for the most, five plunges, suffice to cool the body; in obstinate nervous fevers, however, they are occasionally to be repeated several times in the course of the day. (See Appendix, CC.) There are also

LOCAL BATHS,

by which we understand baths of tepid or cold water, into which a portion of the body is plunged, and in which it remains immersed for a certain time. Their action is more powerful than that of local ablutions.

HEAD BATHS

are used for rheumatic pains in the head, common headaches, rheumatic inflammations of the eye, deafness, loss of smell and taste. They tend to disturb the morbid humors which nature generally evacuates in the form of abscesses in the ears. They are also used to prevent or cure the flow of blood to the head; but in this case only for a few minutes, in order to avoid too great a reaction; and should be followed by exercise in the open air in the shade. This bath is used as follows: a wash hand basin should be placed at the end of a rug on the floor. On this rug the patient should extend himself, so that his head may reach the basin, at the bottom of which may be placed a towel, for the head to rest upon. Then the back of the head must be placed in the water—first on one side and then the other; lastly, the back part of the head is again placed in the water. In chronic inflammations of the eyes, each part of the head should remain in the water for fifteen minutes; and as long for deafness, loss of smell and taste. All this will occupy an hour, during which time the water should be renewed twice. If these baths are continued with perseverance, success is certain. This success is generally announced by violent headache, until the formation of an abscess takes place, which ends by breaking. For the common headaches, the back part of the head may be exposed to the water from ten to fifteen minutes; if they are obstinate, a foot bath and a sitz bath, both slightly chilled, should be used for half an hour each. If necessary, this process may be repeated several times in the course of the day.

THE SITTING BATH

is taken in a vessel or tub so constructed that the patient can remain for the necessary time in a sitting posture; say, from a quarter of an hour to an hour. The bath is made of wood or zinc; the latter is the best. The height of the pedestal of the vessel should be four inches, the diameter seventeen inches, the inner depth nine inches, and the height of the back seven inches. The depth of the water should seldom exceed four inches, in order that the reaction may be the sooner effected. If they produce headache, apply a wet bandage. The best time for using this bath is an hour before dinner, or before going to bed. In the latter case there is the advantage of securing a night's rest to the patient. In order to secure the object sought, the patient should rub the abdomen well with his wet hand or with flannel, and not fail to take exercise in the open air both before and after. If the bath is to act as a stimulant, the water must be very cold, not exceeding 41° of Fahrenheit, two inches deep, and continued for five minutes; where it is to have a tonic action, the temperature should be from 50° to 57° and continued from ten to fifteen minutes. These are to be repeated frequently during the day. This bath is in general use, and of great service in drawing the humors from the head, chest, and abdomen; it relieves flatulency, and is of the utmost value to the sedentary and studious.

FOOT BATHS,

which are employed almost exclusively as a counteracting agent against the pains of the upper part of the body, may be taken in a small tub, at the depth of one or two inches, and continued from fifteen to thirty minutes. When the water becomes warm it should be changed. Care should be taken that the feet are warm before they are put into the water, and exercise should be taken immediately after to bring back the heat to them. Rubbing them with a dry hand assists this very much. Cold foot baths are sure means of preventing tendency to cold feet; the application of hot water only weakens the skin, and renders the feet more susceptible to cold.

THE DROP BATH

is a term applied to the mode of applying single drops of very cold water, which fall from a height of several fathoms, on a particular part of the body, at certain intervals, between which the part is briskly rubbed. It produces violent excitement and irritation of the nervous system; and should not therefore be applied to the vital parts, or such as are abundantly supplied with nerves. They are of great use in chronic cases of paralysis.

THE FINGER BATH

is used for whitlows, etc. The finger is placed in a glass of cold water, three times a day, fifteen minutes each time; the finger and hand bandaged; then the elbow must be placed in water twice a day, and a heating bandage placed on the arm above it; this will have the effect of drawing the inflammation from the hand.

THE LEG BATH

is used when these parts are afflicted with ulcers, ringworms, or fixed rheumatic pains. They act as stimulants, and may be used for an hour, and sometimes longer. They always determine abscesses, and where they already exist, they cause an abundant suppuration.

THE DOUCHE,

of all means employed, is the most powerful in moving bad humors lodged in the system: it is used in the greater number of chronic diseases, and consists of a column of water about the thickness of one's wrist, conducted through a pipe, having a fall of from twelve to twenty feet. This is used with a view to invigorate weak parts, on which the water is made to fall, except the head and chest. It is used from two to ten minutes, and the patient soon becomes delighted with its invigorating effects. The time for douching is one hour after breakfast, and two after dinner; but should never be taken when the body is cold. (See Appendix, DD.) Active exercise should follow and cold water should not be drank immediately after, as a rapid generation of heat is thus impeded. Besides the above, there are the cold bandages, and the stimulating, strengthening, or heating bandages.

THE COLD BANDAGES

have two different operations, each of which is distinct from the other: one is in that of cooling the part to which they are applied, and the other that of raising its temperature. Where the former effects are sought, the cloths should be of a size suited to the part inflamed, folded six or eight times, dipped into very cold water, gently expressed before application, and renewed every five minutes. In cases of inflammation of the brain, etc., the water should not be more than 44°, and should be continued night and day, until danger is averted. One omission of changing the wet cloths at the proper time, will be sufficient to frustrate the beneficial results, for violent reaction is only to be subdued by continued cold. There is no part to which a bandage is so frequently applied as round the body, over the stomach and bowels, for the purpose of increasing the heat of the stomach, and assisting digestion, from which results the formation of better juices. They are applied in an infinity of ways, and are very useful in many complaints; imparting tone to the nerves and vessels of the part to which they are applied. Those afflicted with complaints of the chest and throat, wear one round the neck, and on the breast at night; those with weak and inflamed eyes, wear one at the back of the head and neck; those who have weak digestion and are otherwise debilitated, wear one round the waist all day, while gouty or rheumatic persons have also their feet and legs encased in them by night. The umschlag or bandage is invariably applied to wounds, bruises, and generally diseased parts; as also to any part of the body where pain is felt. Its assuaging power is almost incredible. They cure intestinal congestion, constipation, relaxation, and promote the exuding of bad humors, which is manifest by the color and odors which follow. (Appendix, EE.)

THE HEATING BANDAGES

consist of pieces of linen folded two or three times, and dipped in cold water, well wrung out, and applied to the part; having been drawn lightly round it, a dry bandage is added to prevent, as much as possible, the entrance of cold air. The clothes should be changed only when they begin to dry. These bandages may be worn day and night on any part of the body, and are of great service in any afflictions of the abdomen. In the latter case, take a piece of linen, sufficiently large to go round the body twice, wet one foot of it, or more if necessary; after it has been well wrung out, apply the wet part to the parts affected, which must be covered lightly by the dry parts, twice.

Having thus spoken of the various modes of applying the water, we may proceed to a few of the diseases which are curable by these methods; at the same time reminding our readers that we only throw out hints. First, because we deem prevention better than cure, and therefore beg to refer them to Chapter II., and in most cases little else will be needful; and secondly, our limits being circumscribed, we cannot go into lengthened detail; but if our readers have money to purchase, time to read, mind to comprehend, and stand in need of more minute detail, they may possess it by procuring the "Hand Book of Hydropathy," etc., and a medical dictionary.

The cases treated successfully by this mode are

CONSTIPATION OR COSTIVENESS,

which has been properly denominated "the mother of most chronic diseases;" and those who are afflicted by it are said to "repose on a volcano, the devastating eruption of which is always to be dreaded."

Common sense teaches us that if the alimentary canal becomes closed at the lower extremities, health must be ruined;

as it induces disordered stomachs, depraved appetites, and impaired digestion. These preclude a sufficient supply of nourishment, hence, paleness, laxity, flaccidity, the nervous symptoms, wasting of the muscular flesh, languor, debility, the relaxation of the menses, the suspension of other excretions, serous effusions, dropsy, and death.

The usual modes of combating this evil are the most irrational and unsuccessful; in fact they only tend to strengthen and perpetuate it. Hence it is impossible to describe the horrors produced by Morrison's and Parr's pills, and other purgatives, which have been taken by wholesale. These and all other unnatural and violent stimulants force on an unwilling action, and produce a temporary and deceitful calm, but reaction of a most prejudicial kind succeeds, and a terrible storm, which convulses the whole system, follows. And yet people cannot be persuaded that this habit of swallowing forcing medicines is the chief cause of all their sufferings, both of mind and body. And here let it be distinctly understood, that the evil is not so much in the medicine as in the purging—the effect produced, not the agent which produces it. (See Appendix, FF.)

To prevent or cure constipation, the hydropathic treatment is more successful than any other yet attempted. But the greatest difficulty is in getting people to be firm and patient. They wish to realize effects in a few days which can only be brought about in months; for it will often be found necessary to pursue the treatment for six or twelve months before the bowels will be brought to act naturally. But surely the boon is worth an effort, even a protracted one. The first matters to be attended to are, diet and exercise: let the patient, therefore, read again the chapters on these subjects. Let him then commence in earnest, by rising early in the morning, sponge and rub himself well all over; drink freely of cold water, and take a brisk walk of three or four miles, or use other exercise for an hour, so as to produce a glow of heat. When the costiveness has been of several years standing, add sitz and foot baths, umschlags by day and night, and douches on the abdomen, to correct the weakness of this part. He will find this plan far more effectual than all the tonic, aperient, and antibilious pills and potions, the announcement of which, and of their right honorable, and right reverend patrons, the advertising columns of newspapers and magazines are filled. This treatment has never failed to effect a cure, even in cases where there has been no natural evacuations from the bowels for upward of thirty years.

FEVERS

are of such frequent occurrence, that one half of mankind is said to perish by them alone; but they have invariably yielded to the cold-water treatment; so that of the thousands so treated by Priessnitz, he is said never to have lost a patient in fever. The general symptoms of this disease are increased heat, affections of the head and loins, weariness of the limbs, rigors in various degrees, from shivering to chronic spasms; the nails and lips are livid, and the skin is usually pale, cold, and dry, and the thirst is excessive. (See Appendix, GG.)

During the treatment of fever the patient must abstain from animal food, cheese, eggs, butter, and all stimulating food or drink. His food should be cold. He should drink nothing but cold water. The room must be well aired and dry. All excitement be avoided, and evacuation secured daily. He should lie on a mattrass, sleep as much as possible, and should never be waked under any circumstances.

In the excitement of fever of any kind, the wet sheet, and cold or tepid ablutions are of the first importance. They speedily carry off the morbid heat, relieve pain, and tranquilize the pulse without in any degree adding to the debility of the various structures of the body, already sufficiently great. The propriety of drinking cold water also in fever is clearly indicated, and has proved most beneficial. Instances have occurred at Graefenburg, of persons being kept in the half bath for nine or ten hours, and others being put in from forty to fifty wet sheets in the course of twenty-four hours, with complete success. In the first appearance of fever, let the patient be wrapped in wet sheets, and let umschlags be applied to the head at the same time. The latter are to be charged more frequently than the former, where there is violent headache. The sheets must be repeated according to the degree of fever, every half hour or hour. If the patient be relieved after three or four applications, and his head be clearer, he may be washed with cold water, of about 55°; after which he should take moderate exercise in his room, or if fine, in the open air. Thirst should at all times be relieved by cold water, but during the process of sweating, not so as to check it. During the whole process, the bowels should be kept open by bandages round the body, and by clysters, repeated seven or eight times a day, if necessary; in short, they must be continued till an evacuation is effected. The bandages are not to be renewed before they are perfectly dry.

GOUT

is a formidable monster which appears in various shapes, the medical treatment of which is an act of insanity. Drugs are of no use here; nay, they are injurious. Drs. Mudie and Bigel assert, with a perfect knowledge of causes, and a deep conviction, founded upon innumerable and notable facts, that the sudorific process, and cold water, are the only means of curing this disease. The cure of the gout requires the application of the whole treatment. It should be felt on the entire system, before it be particularly applied to the parts afflicted. (See Appendix, HH.) The first object should be, by the sudorific process, or baths, to relieve that excessive irritability of the skin, which is the source of so much pain; adding to this, exercise in the open air. By degrees gouty subjects should leave off flannel, which they may do with impunity on the fifth or eighth day after treatment. When the patient is not too weak, he may go immediately to the douche, taken generally over the body, but only for a few minutes. It is only when he is able to sustain it easily that he should expose the suffering part to it, to put the humors which are there established, in motion. Cold water must be taken freely; the diet must be vegetable and scanty; much exercise in the open air, and friction, by rubbing and brushing the whole body, and of the affected parts particularly, are very necessary. If the patient be young and strong, much perspiration is of the greatest importance, but with umschlags applied to the diseased parts. Few pass more than five or six weeks under the treatment without having the crisis, i. e., without being charged with eruptions or boils. On the appearance of the crisis, the douche, and process of perspiring, should be either moderated or remitted, in order not to augment the crisis. All that has been said above on gout and its treatment, equally applies to

RHEUMATISM,

which bears such a great resemblance to it, that it is supposed to take the same origin. The principal means to be employed are the application of the wet sheets the first thing in the morning; the next morning sweating in the blankets; the third morning wet sheets again, then the blankets, and so on alternately. After each, a cold ablution; a sitz bath daily at twelve o'clock, and a tepid one at six in the evening, with wet bandages over the painful parts.

INFLAMMATIONS

are very numerous, and arise from various causes.

INFLAMMATION OF THE BRAIN

is the most dangerous, and may prove fatal. The general symptoms are—pain of the head, redness of the eyes, deafness, flushed face, singing in the ears, and intolerance of the light. The patient is noisy, and evinces great strength; has a hard pulse and a hot, dry skin. The treatment should be as follows: The part of the head affected should be shaven immediately, and application of cold water laid over the whole head, and changed every five minutes, or sooner if the bandages become warm; as much depends upon this point. Several napkins should be placed in very cold water, under 40°, if possible, and never above 50°, that the applications may follow in quick succession. To neglect this may be fatal. Sometimes there is great difficulty in getting the patient to drink, as they dislike water; but this must be overcome, if possible. It is also of great importance that the bowels act freely. The head should be raised, the room kept quiet and well aired, and the light excluded. (See Appendix, II.) If after twenty-four hours no favorable symptoms appear—such as free perspiration, copious discharge of blood from the nose, the bleeding piles, plentiful discharge of urine, it is advisable to pour cold water over the whole body of the patient, and by the wet sheets and blankets seek to promote perspiration. If the patient be delirious, the nervous excitement must be allayed by cold affusions, not only of the head, but of the whole body. There are also inflammations of the throat, such as

CROUP;

which dangerous disease is confined to a definite period of infancy, from two to the sixth or eighth year, and takes place in spring generally, or late in autumn. Plethoric children are most endangered by it. The premonitory symptoms are—hoarseness and fretfulness toward evening; to this is added a dry, hollow cough, pulse hard, and the face flushed. As soon as the least of the above symptoms appear, the child should be wrapped in a well wrung wet sheet, and the umschlag applied round its throat, for the purpose of producing perspiration; if the object be promoted, the patient be relieved, the cough loosened, and respiration become more free, he should be allowed to remain at least eight or ten hours in moderate perspiration. This should be followed by an ablution of cold water, at 65 to 70°, when the patient should be put to bed and lightly covered, to keep up a slight action of the skin. As the disease is sometimes of a very insidious character, and may return after all danger was thought to be passed, it is proper to wrap the patient again in wet sheets in the evening, even when he had passed the day favorably, and to renew the applications to the throat, followed by the ablution. For

COMMON SORE THROAT, STIFF NECK, ETC.,

gargle well and often with cold water; rub the throat and chest several times a day with the hand dipped in cold water; and wear a heating bandage round the neck and on the chest, during the night. In some few stubborn cases the wet sheet is necessary, but generally the above will be quite sufficient.

INFLAMMATION OF THE LUNGS

commences, for the most part, suddenly, with a violent rigor, followed by heat, pain in the chest, shortness of breath, restlessness, palpitation of the heart, determination of blood to the head, and may be classed among the most dangerous diseases. It is therefore advisable that some one well versed in the water cure be consulted, if possible. Till this can be accomplished, the patient may be wrapped in a well wrung sheet, a wet bandage (less wrung out) should be applied to his chest, and he should be laid in bed, with his head raised; water may be given him from time to time of 64°. This temperature is best obtained by placing a bottle containing water, well closed, into hot water. If there be a dryness and heat of the skin, the sheets should be changed in half an hour or an hour. The tepid bath must always follow each sweating. The reappearance of a discharge of blood is a very favorable symptom, and should be moderately promoted. (See Appendix, JJ.)

INFLAMMATION OF THE STOMACH

is attended with fixed pains and burning heat in the stomach, nausea and sickness, pulse hard, cold, clammy sweats, and pain upon taking any kind of food. To cure it the patient should take a half bath at 77°, the water of which reaches above the stomach. During the bath he should drink water in small doses (which has stood); but frequently while in the bath his whole body should be washed and gently rubbed by two attendants. The patient should rub the region of the stomach himself as he can bear it. If the particular pain be somewhat abated after the lapse of a quarter of an hour, and the attack be modified, the patient should be conveyed to bed, wrapped in a wet sheet, having previously applied a moderately wrung bandage over his stomach. When this becomes irksome to him, let him take a tepid ablution, apply well wrung bandages round his body; return him to bed, and regulate his covering so that he may be rather warm than cold. Here also obtain help if possible.

INFLAMMATION OF THE BOWELS

is another of its dangerous forms, and is attended with burning pain in the vicinity of the seat of inflammation, which subsequently spreads over the whole abdomen, and produces great heat. This is often succeeded by vomiting, convulsions, and fever. If it arises from a rupture, it should be immediately reduced by an experienced person, if possible, if it will not yield to very cold bandages. Success is sometimes obtained by means of baths of 91°, in which the patient remains for an hour or longer, when he may be able to return the rupture himself. When the inflammation originates in cold, it should be combated at first by clysters of moderately cold water, and by well wrung cloths applied to the whole abdomen, by covering the body sufficiently, and drinking water in small quantities, but frequently.

INFLAMMATION OF THE LIVER

is generally characterized by acute pain below the ribs on the right side, at the same time the part is very sensitive to the touch; the pain is increased by stretching out the arm or leg, also by taking a deep inspiration; in fact, the whole of the right side more or less feels the pain. (See Appendix, KK.) In all diseases, but this particularly, beware of mercury, and have recourse to cold ablutions every morning, with friction; wear the stimulating bandages; take a sitz bath two hours before dinner, and drink cold water freely, with exercise in the open air. The sudorific blankets should be used once or twice a week, or perhaps oftener, as the object should be to promote skin crisis. Dr. Weiss speaks of one of his patients passing a remarkably round gall stone, half an inch in diameter, and rather more in length, as the result of the water treatment—a proof of its efficacy.

INFLAMMATION OF THE KIDNEYS

is attended with sharp pain about the region of the kidneys, which is increased by coughing and vomiting, causing numbness in the thigh of the affected side, and an inability to stand or walk. The patient lies with most ease on the side affected. The urine is generally voided by drops, and sometimes totally suspended. In the treatment, the wet sheets are to be repeated more or less frequently, according to the degree of inflammation; the same applies to the wet bandages, which should not be well wrung out, and changed every five or seven minutes, in severe cases. Cold water should be taken frequently, in small quantities, and clysters and sitz baths are of great service; but the water should be tepid at first.

INFLAMMATORY ERUPTIONS,

or breaking out on the skin, require little more than dietetic treatment, cleanliness, pure air, vegetable food, and nature's beverage, to which may be added, if needed, the wet sheets. The greatest caution becomes necessary to avoid such trash as "Gowland's lotion," etc., etc., all of which tend to check, and throw the eruption inward, instead of enticing it to the surface of the skin. Thousands have been sacrificed in this manner. (See Appendix, LL.)

ERYSIPELAS

attacks chiefly the face and legs, but may present itself on any part of the body. It is often an effort of nature to relieve itself of a dangerous humor by the skin, and should not be submitted immediately to cold ablutions. The entire body should be subjected to the cure. Cold water should be taken frequently, in small doses; the invalid should perspire in a wet sheet, and apply heating bandages to the diseased parts. Care must be taken that the patient does not change the bandages too often, as they are apt to do, with a view of easing the pain; for, although every fresh application brings immediate relief, yet in this manner the exhalation from the skin, which is most essential to recovery, might be easily interrupted. The great object should be to force a crisis of the skin quickly, and when ablutions are used, they should be tepid at first. This treatment, which excludes all cold water ablutions, is always successful, whereas no other is.

MEASLES, SMALL-POX, AND SCARLETINA

are so well known as to need no description. The fever, which generally attends them, constitutes their chief danger. It is its violence which closes the pores, and prevents the breaking out of the eruptive matters, which would give general relief. Directly it is observed, the patient should be wrapped up in a wet sheet, which should be renewed when it becomes warm, if the fever be virulent; but must not be carried too far, so as to interfere with the development of the eruption. The body should not be washed in cold water, but slightly tepid. Congestions of the head and lungs should be combated by cooling applications, and the bowels kept regular by tepid clysters.

DROPSY

is one of those diseases, the cure of which, even by hydropathy, can only be effected under certain conditions. The great object is to produce a crisis by copious sweating, or copious discharge of urine. Before enveloping the patient in the wet sheet, the parts which are swollen, or the whole body, if the dropsy be general, should be well rubbed, for ten minutes, with a rough cloth, or horse-hair gloves. Provide the patient with a urinal when put in the sheet, and allow him to perspire as much as his constitution will bear—the more the better. As to persons being in danger of dropsy from water drinking, the idea is perfectly ridiculous: a case of the kind was never known, and we are persuaded never will be.

ULCERS

require no other treatment than the bandages and the sweating process, under which, we must not be surprised at seeing them enlarge. If, however, this aggravation proceeds too far, the bandage must be dry, and the wounds must be bathed afterward in lukewarm water.

CHOLERA,

which Dr. T. G. Graham says can only be treated successfully by "warmth, opium, and salt," and to which "hydropathy is not at all applicable, has, however, been cured repeatedly by it, and by it alone. Its symptoms are general weariness, flatulency, nausea, a sense of oppression at the stomach, violent purging and vomiting, and constant desire to go to the water closet. The treatment should be a sitz bath, of the temperature of 62°; and if there be headache, apply wet bandages.

Let two or three persons be employed in constantly rubbing the stomach, abdomen, back, legs, and arms, with the hands frequently dipped in cold water, till the natural warmth is produced. In no cases is it so necessary to drink freely of cold water. Cases have occurred in which from twenty to thirty glasses have been taken in an hour. (See Appendix, MM.)

CANCER

is thought to be incurable by water, but only by those who are unacquainted with its efficacy. The treatment is the same as for ulcers, with the exception of the patient perspiring for a longer period every day.

DIARRHŒA (OR LOOSENESS),

when recent, may be successfully treated by drinking freely of cold water, and by taking wet bandages, light food, and sitz baths. It is often an effort of nature to carry off prejudicial humors, which must not be checked, but rather promoted, at least for a time. Those who are subject to attacks of this disorder should take daily ablutions, sitz baths of short duration, adhere to a vegetable diet, and to nature's beverage.

BLEEDING AT THE NOSE

should be met with washing the throat and nape of the neck with cold water, applying a wet bandage to the stomach, or washing the whole body in cold water. (See Appendix, NN.) The colder the water, the better. If the above does not succeed, take a wet sheet, slightly wrung out, folded up in part, lay it on the floor (in summer on a stone floor), and lay the patient on it, with his head rather raised on the sheet, which is now to be wrapped round his body. Cold bandages are at the same time to be applied to his neck and chest, and he is to be lightly covered. This has never failed.

SPITTING OF BLOOD

is not always to be considered as a primary disease. It is often only a symptom, and, in some cases, not an unfavorable one. This is the case in pleurisies, etc. In the dropsy, scurvy, or consumption it is a bad symptom, and shows that the lungs are ulcerated. The treatment of this disease, especially if it be far advanced, is very difficult, and requires great caution; therefore, none should attempt it but those well versed in the art. The same remarks will apply to

VOMITING OF BLOOD,

which is equally, if not more dangerous than the preceding; the treatment of which, as also that of uterine flooding, mucous discharges, etc., are described with great minuteness in the able work of Mr. Weiss; but his remarks are too extensive for our limits.

DYSENTERY

is generally occasioned by indulgence in unripe fruit, sleeping at night with open windows, etc., and is considered contagious. The symptoms are much like those of diarrhœa, and also the mode of treatment. The symptoms however differ, in that there is more acute pain of the bowels, blood generally appears in the stools, to which when the patient goes he feels a bearing down, as if the whole bowels were falling out; and sometimes a part of the intestines is actually protruded. At the commencement of the attack, the patient should drink cold water copiously, at short intervals; and clysters should be used, at first tepid, afterward of cold water; and after the bowels are completely emptied of their contents, copious perspiration must be promoted.

COMMON COLDS—COUGH.

Nothing is more common than to hear people cry, "Beware

that you do not take cold!" But we never hear them cautioned against taking heat. They become as delicate about facing a little cold, and proceed as cautiously as if they were conscious they were walking on the brink of some precipice; but you may keep frizzling them in the heat till they are almost baked, and no concern is manifested. But the fact is, we ought to be more afraid of taking heat, for that will be much more prejudicial to our health than cold. Small as may be the notice taken of these complaints at first, they are often of fearful consequence, as laying the foundation of various other disorders. They chiefly arise from obstructed perspiration, or having previously taken heat. The great object should be to increase the tone of the nerves, and avoid every thing calculated to lessen it. Heat generally lowers it, while cold, wisely applied, at proper times, and in due degrees, heightens it. The moment that tone is given, it causes an invigorated action of the vessels, which insures an improved secretion and excretion, whereby irritation and pain are always relieved, and the way paved for restoration. Here then we recognize, at once, the mode of action of the invaluable agency of cold water, and find a full and sufficient answer to many of the objections advanced against the practice of hydriatics. Great attention should be paid to the state of the skin; the patient should drink freely of cold water, and be much in the open air. If he has cough only, let him gargle well with cold water; rub the throat and chest several times a day with the hand dipped in cold water; wear a heating bandage round the neck and on the chest at night.

PAIN AT THE CHEST

is treated the same as the gout, which has been previously described.

SORE EYES.

When the eye has been injured by external means, first remove the cause, as far as possible, after which make use of the external and internal application of water in the best form adapted to the case. Where it arises from the state of the body, it must not be treated locally only, but generally. In some cases the back of the head should be placed in cold water three times a day, for ten minutes each time, and the eye bath be used for five minutes, twice a day. After the eyes are closed in water for about a minute, they should be opened for the other four minutes. At night apply a heating bandage at the back of the neck; this, and also the head bath, have a tendency to draw all inflammation from the front part of the head. In most cases foot baths twice a day are highly beneficial.

WOUNDS.

Keep the wounded part in tepid water until it ceases bleeding, then put on a heating bandage; when this becomes warm, put another larger one over it, so that it may extend beyond the part afflicted. If the foot be wounded, let it remain in the water for an hour twice a day, to draw out the inflammation; then apply the bandage night and day, but continue it far beyond the wounded part.

NOSE COLDS,

when not of long continuance, are considered healthy as relieving the system of some of the bad humors. To cure this, snuff cold water up the nostrils several times a day, be much in the open air, and wear a heating bandage on the forehead at night. To cure

BURNS,

apply constantly to the part cold wet cloths, without a dry one over them.

DEAFNESS

should be treated by rubbing the body all over twice a day with a cold wet cloth, wearing a heating bandage over the ears at night, and drinking plentifully of cold water. This process will very often relieve deafness, but in obstinate cases the whole treatment must be resorted to.

ASTHMA.

The triumphs of hydropathy in the cure of asthma have been very great, chiefly by invigorating the digestive organs, and the whole frame, and not by virtue of any specific influence on the respiratory apparatus. Though in this respect great relief has sometimes been afforded. T. R——, of U——, had been a great sufferer from asthma, and after one week's abstinence from drugs, hot liquids, and animal food, and by drinking thirty glasses of cold water a day, taking a daily ablution with much friction, and as much exercise in the open air as he could bear, he threw up a solid mass of phlegm nearly the size of his hand; of course he was instantly relieved. He continued improving upon the above plan, with an occasional wet sheet, till, at the end of five weeks, he found his appetite returned—his strength greatly increased—his breath nearly as good as ever it was—and he had gained nine pounds in weight. Constant exercise in pure air, combined with a vegetable diet, cold ablutions, sweating, the abandonment of flannel, the plunge bath, douche, etc., work so great an improvement in the digestive organs and chest, as perfectly to rid the sufferer of this very troublesome complaint. As this is not properly an affection of the lungs, but of the stomach and intestines, the digestive organs are its grand and primary seat. It is therefore, as Dr. Graham observes, necessary in some obstinate cases to confine the patient to so small a quantity of food, that he will at times almost be disposed to devour his fingers' ends. The patient should drink cold water plentifully, avoid stimulating food, eat no suppers, walk much up hill, in order to bring the lungs into full play, sweat in the wet sheet every second day, followed by a cold ablution, to which may be added a shallow foot bath for five minutes, just before returning to bed, to be followed by rubbing with a rough cloth, until they are quite warm. Friction between the shoulders and on the chest is of great service, which sometimes produces boils, and which should be encouraged for a time. Many cases of instantaneous relief have been witnessed, by administering cold water only in

SICKNESS OR VOMITING.

We refer to one or two. The wife of the Rev. J. Howell, of Brill, was suddenly seized with incessant sickness. Her medical attendant administered brandy, port wine, tea, etc., all of which were instantly ejected, which induced him to say she could not survive long. She begged for a cup of cold water, which he refused; but through the interference of several teetotalers, and at the request of her husband, he consented: she at once revived; more was given to her with good effect, and she was soon pronounced out of danger. Also, James Osborne, of Berkhamstead, became ill, with loss of appetite, and constant sickness. Nothing would stay on his stomach except cold water, which soon placed him out of danger. Many other cases might be called, showing that "water is best."

TIC DOLOUREUX

is a very painful, and in some cases, a very obstinate disease, of a rheumatic, gouty, or nervous character; is very irregular in its invasion and course; and is one of those diseases given up by the doctor, as well as by the patient. Yet, under the water treatment, cases have occurred of relief being afforded in two hours, and a thorough cure effected in a few days, while the disease has been only acute. Where it is of long standing, and chronic, it is not so easily dealt with. When it is occasioned by a cold, the object should be to incite a crisis by perspiration, or in some other way, by means of the envelopment and cold ablutions. As every thing depends upon a crisis, every thing possible should be done to produce it. If the disease be chronic, great attention should be paid to diet, which should be vegetable. Most cases will yield to a vegetable diet, heating bandages, proper potations of cold-water clysters, and sitz baths.

PART VII.

CHAPTER XII.

PROGRESSIVE REFORM.—MISCELLANEOUS AND CONCLUDING REMARKS.

To remain half way is a useless labor; in all things we must go right to the end.—D'AUBIGNE.

"It is seldom that any combination of men is limited to its original elements, or its proposed object. There is a gravitation in the social, as well as in the physical world."

"Give me one hundred teetotalers, who are anxious only to know, and to diffuse the truth, rather than ten thousand who are disposed to be quiet, and to keep back part of the truth." "The truth, the whole truth, and nothing but the truth." "It is more noble to head our age, than to be in its rear."

ONE of the greatest evils from which mankind have suffered, and are still suffering, is, that they have allowed custom and appetite to be their teachers and rulers, instead of reason, observation, facts, and revelation. Hence many noble efforts, made to remove the various social, physical, and moral evils under which mankind are groaning, have been rendered nugatory. This unhappy influence has crept in among some of our temperance reformers, and has considerably retarded the full development of our glorious principles. We have before endeavored to show that this progressive reform for which we plead, is only carrying out the principle of the temperance reformation; hence, we can only account for the conduct and fears of some of our friends, on the ground that there are among us three classes of individuals, consisting of men *behind* their day—men *before* their day—and men *of* their day. There are men behind their day, and in some respects men behind themselves, for in other matters, they are among the leaders. Here, however, they hang as dead weights upon the energies of their more advanced brethren, and seem exceedingly conscious of alarm at every onward movement: they feel as little sympathy with their times, as their times feel with them. Their cry is, "You go too fast and too far; the people are not ready for your extreme views." Perhaps not, and we question if they ever will be, if left to you and to themselves. But we rejoice to know, there are men who are before their day, though their number is but few; nor is it, perhaps, to be expected, that they should be numerous, though the duties they have to perform, are something like the ancient prophets: pointing to the future, and preparing the people for its arrival. Standing on a loftier eminence than their cotemporaries, their eye sweeps along the horizon; and though the distant cloud is no larger than a man's hand, they regard it as the precursor of a glorious rain, and it enables them to speak of subjects, and to promise blessings, which sound strange to the multitude. Nevertheless, their voice is being heard, and we trust shall never cease to be heard in the world, correcting its abuses, exalting its views, animating its activity, enlarging its expectations, and enhancing its real happiness. There are also men of their day, who, marking its peculiarities, and falling in with its movements, accelerate its progress toward a better state of things: of these there are thousands engaged in the temperance cause, whose conduct does great credit to their heads and to their hearts. They have learned one great point, to "cease to do evil," by having been taught to abandon a physical poison, and now they are going on, in a physical sense, to "learn to do well" in other respects. They have adopted Brother Jonathan's motto—"Get right, and go ahead!" They have got right in reference to alcoholic drinks, and now they are going ahead to destroy other baneful customs and practices. And why should they be satisfied with pulling down the temple of Bacchus, magnificent though the achievement be ; let them go on, and "take us the foxes, the little foxes, that spoil the vines: for our vines have tender grapes." Let the formation of correct habits, as far as possible, be promoted with regard to food, drink, cleanliness, air, exercise, drugs, water, etc., and the health and longevity, the happiness, ay, and the salvation of the community will be promoted thereby.

This subject has been treated with some ability by "Berean," in the "Temperance Weekly Journal," a high water mark paper, which ought to be read by all. In reference to the use of tea, coffee, tobacco, etc., he says, "Why, unquestionably, if a man knowingly uses that which is physically injurious, he commits moral evil. Yea, if he wastes, on that which is merely worthless, money which ought to be employed in doing good, then, unquestionably, he is morally guilty. 'To him that knoweth to do good, and doeth it not, to him it is sin.'

"Perhaps," says he, "I may be allowed to give a few reasons why I think the pledged abstainer from alcohol will do well to discountenance all other injurious articles of food and drink.

"1. One artificial, injurious custom has a natural tendency to support another, therefore tobacco smoking will support alcohol drinking.

"2. It cannot be expected that the slave of one bad habit can be the most efficient reformer of customs and usages near akin to that by which he himself is enslaved.

"3. If the same physical laws which declare alcohol to be a poison, also declare tea, coffee, tobacco, etc., to be poisons, then the man who urges those laws in support of abstinence from the former poisons, will, at all events, not be in any degree the less consistent if he also urges the same laws in support of abstinence from the latter poisons.

"4. There may be cases in which a thorough-going reformer may consider it expedient to avoid attacking several bad usages at once, but very often that which appears to superficial observers to be expedient, is, in the end, found to be very bad policy. Sound principle and sound expediency always go together; etc.

"5. It is the soundest policy, and, therefore, the most expedient, in carrying out the principles on which the temperance reformation is based, to keep well in advance of public opinion, until public opinion is brought up to the standard of truth. By keeping far in advance of public opinion, we keep up an interest in our advocacy, arising from the very opposition which that advocacy excites, providing that opposition is an opposition referring to the principles of our cause, and not founded on personal animosities, or of party spirit.

"6. Abstinence from alcohol, opium, tobacco, tea, coffee, mustard, pepper,* mint, sage, onions [animal food], and all similar exciting and strongly flavored articles is much more in advance of public opinion than mere abstinence from alcoholic liquors; and, consequently, if such comprehensive abstinence is founded on the principles of truth, it will, whenever it is advocated with equal ability and zeal, create much more public interest, and will prove much more efficient than mere abstinence from alcohol. It will lead people to take more enlarged and comprehensive views of the great temperance question. They will be more impressed with its magnitude and importance, and their zeal to exert themselves in its favor will be excited in a corresponding degree. The more I study this great question, the more convinced I am, that in reference to it, in all its various bearings, it is our duty to abandon the principle of slavish expediency, and to be only anxious to promote the inquiry, and the solution of the inquiry—'What is truth?'"

Condiments, particularly those of the spicy kind, are non-essential to the process of digestion, in a healthy state of the system. They afford no nutrition. Though they may assist the action of a debilitated stomach, for a time, their continual use never fails to produce an indirect debility of that organ. They affect it as alcohol or other stimulants do. The present

* The English consume about six millions pounds of pepper annually.

relief afforded, is at the expense of future suffering.—*Dr. Beaumont.* Besides which, they induce us to eat more than nature requires, for which end they are taken. A gracious Providence gave them to the Indians, because their burning sun enervates their bodies, which then require stimulants. In our climate, on the contrary, the air is more compressed, and, consequently, contains more oxygen, which predisposes us to take in inflammatory diseases; stimulants, therefore, only augment this predisposition. Let us use, says Priessnitz, seasonings which nature has given us, and leave foreigners to theirs. (See Appendix, OO.)

As to people not being able to do without tea, coffee, tobacco, etc., the idea is perfectly ridiculous. How did our ancestors do without them? Tea has not been imported into Europe 200 years; and even then, not as a beverage, but for medicinal purposes. It was first used in Britain about the year 1666; and became a fashionable beverage at court, owing to the example of Katherine, queen of Charles II., who had been accustomed to it in Portugal.

Some of the most respectable authorities that modern medicine can produce, have strongly condemned the use of tea; among whom are Cullen, Tissot, Linnæus Kæmpfer, Curry, Beaumont, etc. They object to the use of tea, because, 1., the tea leaf, when fresh from the tree, is of a poisonous nature, and though it loses some of its acrimony, by its being steeped, and afterward dried, yet, even in that state, in which it is sent to this country, it retains much of its narcotic or stupifying qualities. 2. There is an astringency in tea which renders it extremely injurious to the constitution, and like the frequent bracing of a drum, must ultimately relax and debilitate. 3. In addition to its natural pernicious qualities, the manner in which it is prepared, by being dried either on iron or copper plates, must ultimately be extremely injurious. The corrosions of copper are undoubtedly pernicious; those of iron may not perhaps, be equally so, yet the effluvia of any steaming metal cannot be favorable to health. 4. The manner in which teas are conveyed to Europe, closely packed up in slight wooden chests, lined with a composition of lead and tin, and liable to be affected by the corrosion of those two metals, must render the article here much more unwholesome than even in China. 5. Not only is the tea itself a pernicious article, but it is often mixed with a variety of other substances, of an injurious character, with a view, it is said, to improve its color or flavor. 6. Its evil effects are increased by its being taken hot. All hot liquids enfeeble the digestive organs, the stomach, and the alimentary canal; are not so easily and readily absorbed by the lymphatic vessels, and do not promote the circulation so well as cold water.

Dr. Duncan, in his "Treatise on Hot Liquors," says, That by hot liquors, the blood is inflamed; and such whose blood is inflamed, live not so long as those who are of a cooler temper; a hot blood being commonly the cause of fluxes, rheums, ill-digestion, pains in the limbs, headache, dimness of sight, and especially of hysteric vapors. He also imputes the cause of ulcers to a hot blood, and declares that if men keep their blood cool and sweet, by a moderate and cooling diet, they would never be troubled with ulcers, or any breakings out.

Dr. Millingen, in his "Curiosities of Medical Experience," tells us he "knew a person who could never never indulge in tea without experiencing a disposition to commit suicide, and nothing could arouse him from this state of morbid excitement but the pleasure of destroying something—books, papers, or any thing within his reach. Under no other circumstance than this influence of tea were these fearful aberrations observed."

Dr. F. Lee, editor of the "National Temperance Advocate," being asked what was the best beverage for morning and evening repasts, said, "Beyond all question, water is the proper beverage of man."

Dr. Harris says, Tea has injured thousands annually, by affecting the nerves, disturbing the functions of the brain, weakening the coats of the stomach, and otherwise enfeebling the digestive organs, as well as destroying the healthy hue of blooming and youthful faces. How many wrinked old maids are to be met with throughout her majesty's dominions, who have made themselves look aged and wrinkled by the imprudent use of tea, with all its adulterations; etc.

R. T. Claridge, Esq., says, If the female portion of the community knew how injurious these drinks were, principally because they are taken hot; how they spoil the skin, take away its delicacy, render it rough and yellow, and consequently cause them to lose, before their time, their freshness of complexion, the color of their cheeks, the coral hue of the lips, the whiteness of the teeth, and the brilliancy of the eyes, so as to imprint on the physiognomy the traces of premature old age; these reasons would, I am persuaded, be sufficient to occasion them to renounce these beverages, and drink only cold water; a resolution which would guarantee them against these losses, and preserve to them, as long as possible, the charms of their sex.

Professor Liebig asserts, that coffee impedes the digestion of food for an hour or two, its carbonaceous principle requiring oxygen; and that green tea should be looked upon as a poison.

Dr. Graham, of America, declares that there is no truth in science more perfectly demonstrable than that alcohol is one of the most energetic and fatal poisons known to man; and with equal certainty can it be proved that tea, coffee, tobacco, and opium are powerful poisons to the human body.

Dr. Graham says, "Formerly I ranged myself among those who looked upon black tea as a wholesome beverage; but among the many changes which time, observation, and reflection have wrought in my sentiments, this is one, that we had better let tea alone! I think it weakens the stomach, etc."

Mr. Whitlaw says, "The next destructive drink of which I have to take notice, is tea. To persons 'whose anxious inquiry is the way to health,' I would say, avoid the use of tea. If the digestive organs be weak, and the body otherwise predisposed to disease, the effects of tea on the system is most injurious. It may, indeed, be a slow poison, as I have often been told; but at the same time, it is a certain one. That class of diseases commonly called nervous, tremors, habitual depression of spirits, and all the miserable train of symptoms arising from laxity and debility, may justly be ascribed, in nine cases out of ten, to this insidious poison. Even its moderate use gives rise to many distressing symptoms, such as flatulency, a sensation of sinking at the stomach, watchfulness, and the feeble tremulousness known by the epithet *nervous*."

As Dr. Cullen lived in the age when the injurious effect of tea was beginning to show itself on the constitutions of the people, we will hear his opinion. After referring to the experiments of Drs. Smith and Lettsom, and to "the observations which I have made in the course of fifty years, in all sorts of persons, I am convinced that the qualities of tea are narcotic and sedative." Speaking of the "poisonous nature of tea," he asserts that this does not arise, as "has been alleged," from "the large quantity of warm water which commonly accompanies it;" though he admits "some bad effects may arise from this cause: but from attentive observation, I can assert, that wherever any considerable effects appear, they are in nine of every ten persons entirely from the qualities of the tea; and that any like effects of warm water do not appear in one of a hundred who take in this very largely."

"Cold water! let thy praise be sung by every son of earth;
Yet all the pens of wisest scribes can never tell thy worth:
Thou lucid, sparkling, glitt'ring gem, by mercy thou wert given;
Thy crystal streams refresh our souls, and make us think of heaven."
J. Inwards.

Among the various articles of foreign growth, which a vitiated appetite has introduced into general use, is coffee, which was first known in England about 1652. Perhaps the best thing that can be said of it, is, that it powerfully counteracts the effects of narcotics, and hence it is used by the Turks, with some propriety, in abating the influence of the inordinate quantities of opium they are accustomed to swallow. In proportion as coffee is indulged in, it proves stimulating and heating, creating thirst, and producing watchfulness, tremors, and many of those complaints called nervous; it has a very bad effect on persons subject to bilious attacks and sick headaches. Let such try cold water for breakfast one week, and they will be convinced of the justness of our remarks. We know, to them, it will not be very comfortable, nor can we conceive it very comfortable to be constantly, or nearly so, troubled with sick headache, etc.

As a proof of the bad effects of tea, coffee, etc., let a nervous or dyspeptic person use two or three cups of strong tea, and the effects will be nightmare, disturbed sleep, and the other violent symptoms of indigestion, etc. Coffee will produce fever, disturbed rest, and in the morning, headache and heartburn; the dose is repeated, the excitement which it produces gives an hour's relief, but it only strengthens the cause of their uneasiness, and renders permanent the effects.

Water, cold water, is therefore preferable to artificial, hot drinks, of any kind, because it promotes health—does not injure the nerves—promotes sleep—it is nature's beverage—it is highly nutritious and strengthening—has been recommended by the cream of the medical profession—has been the exclusive drink of most who have been noted for great muscular strength, health, and longevity—and, what is very important, it is the most economical. This latter remark we shall seek to amplify and improve hereafter.

Of the sottish, silly, expensive, and injurious habits of smoking, chewing, and snuffing, we cannot avoid saying a few words. Some have so high an opinion of their moral and physical qualities, that they wonder that Milton, in speaking of the productions of Eden, had never mentioned the noblest of them all, the tobacco plant. This plant, as shown by Dr. A. Clarke, was not, as is generally supposed, introduced into this country by Sir W. Raleigh, but by Mr. R. Lane, some time about 1385. In 1796, the tobacco imported into this kingdom amounted to 23,608,775 lbs. Of this, 11,490,446 lbs. were delivered out for home consumption, the duty of which, paid to government, amounted to £287,252 11*s*.* In two years it had increased so much, that in 1798, seventy ships, laden with this noxious weed, came into the port of London, whose cargoes amounted to 40,000,000 lbs.!

Were it not too serious a matter, we might be almost tempted to smile at the paltry arguments adduced in favor of tobacco, etc. The poor man says, it stays his stomach when he has no food—perhaps it may; but it is only by injuring its powers of digestion. On the other hand, if it stays an empty stomach, the expenditure tends to keep it empty—as well as the stomachs of those who are dependent upon its consumers. The practice also tends to keep schools partially empty as well as stomachs; many not being able to send their children in consequence of this drain of the pocket.

The filthy habit of making a dust hole of the nose† is become so common that one would be almost disposed to think our streets were as famous for bad smells as are those of Edinburgh, and therefore the nostrils are filled with the powder of this dangerous weed, which is called snuff. Foreigners may think these persons mad, but this is a mistake, they are only foolish. "This snuff gives a man something to do when he has nothing; spares many an empty head the trouble of making an answer; gives politicians, hypocrites, and knaves time to compound a lie, when they have not one ready; furnishes a wise look for a fool's face; enables men by grimace to cover an emotion; and prevents people leading you by the nose, for fear of dirtying their fingers;" at least so says "The Commissioner;" and we think he is more than half right. So that after all, as its votaries assert, it is not altogether useless.

* The cost of a hogshead of tobacco, of 1200 lbs., varies from £14 to £25; the duty of which is £198.

† It has been justly remarked that if Providence had designed the nose for a dust hole, he would have turned it the other way upward; and man for a smoking animal, he would have made a hole in the top of his head to answer the purpose of a chimney.

It is really astonishing that this "smoke-plague," in less than 300 years should have spread as it has, justifying the remarks of Quarles, who says,

> "Tobacco! a vanity, that has beset
> The world, and made more slaves than Mahomet;
> That has condemn'd us to the servile yoke
> Of slavery, and made us slaves to smoke."

Teetotalers, as a body of physical reformers, ought not to encourage smoking and snuffing, because the habit is

1. Useless. Not indeed to the government, as it pays a very large duty—nor to the vender, as he makes a good profit; but to the consumer it yields no benefit, but is a constant drain upon his pocket. It does not satisfy the cravings of hunger, by imparting the least portion of nutriment—will not quench thirst—does not enrich him, adorn him, or render him respectable or useful. Quite the reverse. It is emphatically a useless habit. It is

2. Foolish. Of all the habits which men have contracted, smoking is one of the most foolish. To see a man, it may be a man of education, benevolence, and intelligence, calling himself a gentleman, ay, and a Christian too, sticking a pipe or a cigar in his mouth, and drawing in, for the purpose of puffing out, the smoke of a lighted herb, does appear truly ridiculous. The author has induced several old smokers to try to smoke in the dark, which sets the practice in a still more ridiculous light. Few can so enjoy it, and many are not able to tell whether their pipe is in or out.

The following circumstance took place in Liverpool, wherein a reformer of evil habits satirized with good effect. He drank tea with a number of smokers in a celebrated temperance hotel, and insinuated himself into their good graces. The tray being removed, pipes and tobacco were introduced, and had got well to work, when he rang the bell, and desired the waiter to bring a basin with water, some soap, and a clean pipe. With the water and soap he made a lather, and commenced to blow bubbles; he launched them one after another into the air, where they floated for a time like Lilliputian balloons; these burst, and had their places supplied by others newly formed. How the smokers did but laugh at the silly man, who had chosen to adopt such a childish amusement! At their sneers he was evidently chagrined, as he rose from his seat and said: "Gentlemen, you have each chosen your own amusement, I mine; and that blowing bubbles is more rational, more philosophical than smoking tobacco, I am prepared to prove. You draw air through a pipe, I blow air through it—your smoke ascends upward, so do my bubbles; they are much cheaper, much cleanlier, do not pollute the atmosphere, and are withal more philosophical—Sir Isaac Newton blew soap bubbles to ascertain some of the properties of light."

This satire and reasoning had its effect on some, who admitted its force, and never smoked again; while others frowned upon the satirist as a regular spoil-company, as some will no doubt do on us, for devoting so much space to so light a subject as smoke; but this is because they are not alive to the philosophy of smoking. It is

3. Injurious to the producer; hence, since the American war, the culture of this herb has decreased considerably in Virginia, the proprietors of the land finding it more profitable to devote the ground to the produce of corn. They found also that the culture of tobacco impoverished the land, reduced both men and animals to a miserable state of dependence—was very perplexing and laborious—in a word, that it has every kind of inconvenience connected with it. It is injurious to the consumer, both as it respects health and morals, intellect and circumstances. It is a powerful narcotic, and also a strong stimulant, and taken internally, in small doses, proves powerfully emetic and purgative. Its essential oil is celebrated for its extreme virulence, and when applied to a wound is said by Redi, to be as fatal as the poison of a viper.* An eminent

* Dr. A. Clarke says a single drop of the chemical oil of tobacco, put

author says tobacco is a very powerful narcotic poison. If the saliva, the secretion of which it provokes, be impregnated with its essential oil, and so swallowed, the deleterious influence is communicated directly to the stomach; or if, as more frequently happens, it is rejected, then the blandest fluid of the human frame, that which, as a solvent and diluent, performs an office in digestion secondary only to the gastric juice itself, is lost. Kœmpfer ranks it with the strong vegetable poisons. No medical or scientific man of modern date has dared to record in writing an opinion in favor of the practice, but many have against it. It is

4. Vulgar.* Only dwell upon the idea for a few moments. Who are the persons that are the greatest slaves to the habit? Generally the sot, the idle; persons who have little respect for themselves, and are little respected by others—the outcast of society. This consideration alone ought to weigh with respectable people, and induce them to abandon it. It has been said, and pertinently, that the practice of smoking and chewing, and snuffing, was more befitting the negroes of Jamaica, the Hottentots of Africa, and the savage tribes of America, than the enlightened and intellectual inhabitants of Great Britain. Happily, this consideration is beginning to influence some; hence very few use the "vulgar pipe," who can command the more respectable cigar. But then, such fall under the lash, which those deserve who practice a habit so

5. Expensive. Think of five millions of money (some assert seven and a half) spent annually in dust and smoke. Many persons, scarcely able to procure the necessaries of life (some not able), yet by sacrificing health and decency, spend

on a cat's tongue, produced violent convulsions, and killed her in the space of one minute.

* Merchants frequently lay tobacco in log houses, to the end that becoming impregnated with the volatile salt of the excrements, it may be rendered brisker, stronger, and more fœtid. In preparing cigars and twist, and in preserving them, stale urine is used to keep them moist, and to preserve their flavor. Think of this when you smoke and chew tobacco! We can vouch for the above, having been behind the scene.

one shilling and sixpence per week, some more.* But even the former sum amounts to nearly £200 in fifty years, and at compound interest would amount, in fifty years, to £800 sterling. Is it possible for Christians to vindicate such conduct? If so, any thing may be vindicated, on the score of expenditure.

6. Offensive. The author of these pages has, on more than one occasion, been made ill by the fumes of tobacco; so much so as to be obliged to leave the room, notwithstanding he had been a considerable smoker for twelve years. Again, how offensive it is to sit behind a schoolboy, dandy, shopman, or fop, on a stage-coach, puffing away his pipe or cigar. It is true, some few ladies tolerate smoking, but most of them detest it, as well they might. Persons addicted to the use of tobacco are not generally aware how very offensive to others it renders their breath, or they would soon leave it off. Again, how it discolors and injures the teeth! In fact, their parlors, clothes, furniture, etc., are all tainted with the stinking nuisance. Alas! that respectable men should submit to such low, miserable habits. It encourages

7. Slavery. Not only are thousands slaves to the habit, but slave-labor is actually employed to produce this luxury for the freeborn sons of Britain, for Christians, and even for *teetotalers*. Yes, this tobacco is prepared for the social pipe, the friendly pinch, and for the delicious quid, at the expense of a hopeless and interminable slavery to thousands of our fellow-men; and of the whip, the lash, the labor, and the sorrow of a slave. Yes, the sighs and groans of the slave may be heard in every breeze, and may serve to assist to waft indulgence and evil to the shores of our land of liberty. It has, therefore, been said, that every penny spent in tobacco is one farthing premium to perpetual slavery, and to encourage the planters in Cuba and Virginia to buy African slaves to

* Many families spend double this sum—and some treble. If they only spend double, by paying it into the building society, they might live rent free, and in ten years have the house for thier own.

increase slavery. Think of this when you smoke tobacco. It is

8. Demoralizing. An eminent writer on ethics calculates that one tenth of all drunkards are made such by first getting a liking for tobacco. "Over this they talk politics, religion, science, morals, refinement; abuse the government for dishonesty, the people for stupidity, the parsons for hypocrisy, and tradesmen for knavery; and finish, while they blow the last blast in each other's faces, and shake the dust out of the mouth of the instrument, by remarking, 'I'll tell you what, we are in a strange mess altogether.' After this, they send for the ladies, if they have no drawing-room to retire to, and take a cup of tea; having spanned the earth for their afternoon's gratification—the drinks of Asia and Europe, and the smoke of America." And yet some say it does not lead to drinking. Can all this be done without it? We know it is not. After the youngster has learned to smoke, he must go to the pot-house; at first for the sake of company, and then for the sake of the drink. Then he learns to gamble, swear, and fight; and then many have recourse to thieving to support the cost of drinking, smoking, and loss of time. Hear what the Rev. J. A. James says: "It may seem trifling to say, that the first cigar a young man takes within his lips often proves his first step in a career of vice. I grieve and tremble over every youth whom I see contracting this habit; it often leads to other and worse things." Dr. Fothergill says, "The consideration whether or not it is right for Christians* to indulge in the use of tobacco, or to traffic in it, is one of no trifling importance. It is one that is happily claiming a large share of attention, and great good will doubtless result from strict investigation, and free and temperate discussion. My own observation has led me to believe that its ordinary use is a source of great evil, that it is wholly unnecessary, and that its universal abandonment would be highly advantageous."

* The use of tobacco is a criminal indulgence, unbecoming the professors of the wisdom of God.—*Rev. Dr. Hamilton.*

Those who wish to be further informed on this subject, we recommend to read Dr. A. Clarke's "Dissertation on the Use and Abuse of Tobacco," "The Anti-Smoker," "Friendly Advice, etc.," by Ridley.

Hoping we have succeeded in proving that health, enjoyment, and longevity are matters very much under our own control; that animal food, strong drinks, tea, coffee, all hot drinks, tobacco, snuff, etc., are not only useless, but positively hurtful, we shall proceed to show that people use them, not because they are necessary, but because they like them; and that, on the principle of self-denial, and the promotion of the public good, it is the duty of all to abandon them.

Is it not really grievous to think of a rational Christian man, capable of high intellectual, refined, spiritual enjoyment, taking some or all of the above articles, for the same reasons that boys eat sugar-plums, because they like them? Truly, "there is no accounting for taste." It is one of the most artificial things in the world, to gratify which, men will rob themselves of their independence,* and of their means of doing good to the bodies and souls of men. It is possible for men, and even animals, to train themselves to like or dislike any thing. Hence the Esquimaux, who delights in train-oil, candles, and rotten flesh, is disgusted at sugar. The Red Indians eat large quantities of vermin, and even clay; the Chinese regard rats and dogs as delicious fare. The Asiatic wraps up a small portion of quicklime in a betel-leaf, and chews it, as many here chew tobacco; and our more polished neighbors, the French, regard a dish

* It is not the greatness of a man's means that makes him independent, so much as the smallness of his wants; and it is much easier to save than to get money. To do the former, you have only to consult yourself; for the latter, others. How many, by living up to, rather than a little under, their income, have deprived themselves of the last portion of that independence, which ought to be dear to every man! They are, therefore, bound down by their taskmasters, in a state of vassalage. That man only, who lives within his income, can be just, humane, charitable, and independent; while he who lives beyond it becomes, almost necessarily, rapacious, mean, faithless, and contemptible.

of frog-soup as a great dainty. Therefore the argument of the agreeable flavor of an article proves nothing. But in reference to many of our enjoyments, so called, we think we pay "too dear for our whistle." We purchase at too high a price—the price of our consistency, the sacrifice of our health and real enjoyment, and that of the interests of humanity* and religion.

It cannot be consistent for teetotalers and Christians (both of whom profess to be influenced by the principles of self-denial, and a desire to do good to all men, to the utmost possible extent) to spend the vast sums of money they do on

* The use of tea, by the Americans and Europeans, has a fatal effect upon the Chinese. In the first place, the tea-plant takes up a great part of their land, so that they have not sufficient left to grow provisions; and so scarce is land, in some places, that whole streets or towns are built upon rivers, and people live in floating houses all their lives. Then a large portion of their time is taken up in gathering and preparing the tea, so as to leave little for cultivation of the land not so occupied. This loss of land and time produce the same effect on the Chinese as the growth of opium does on the Hindoos. The people have not sufficient to support them even in the best years; and when a partial famine comes, they perish by thousands. Mr. Malcolm, who visited China as a deputation from the American Baptist Missionary Society, represents the condition of the people there as being most deplorable. He says he saw a number of men lying in the market-place dying and dead, from absolute want; and that this was a common thing. The poor people go round begging for bread, so long as they can get any, and then lie down and die; and W. Barrow says that, in one city alone, nine thousand little helpless children are cast out to perish every year, by their own parents, because they have not the means of rearing them. This is the effect which our use of tea has upon the poor Chinese; this is the way in which they live, or rather die, by our use of tea. The opium which the Chinese use is the life and blood of the Hindoo, and the tea which we use is the life and blood of the Chinese. All who use it are accomplices in this robbery and destruction. These remarks are equally applicable to the consumption of coffee, tobacco, snuff, and cigars. The ground and time that are devoted to their growth might be employed in promoting the improvement and well-being of the whole human family. This has been urged by anti-teetotalers. We cannot say they are necessaries. Then give them up. (See more on this subject, in "Temperance and Luxury," by Pasco.)

tea,* coffee,† tobacco,‡ etc., while their societies are crippled for want of funds; drunkards dying by thousands; and sinners going to hell by multitudes. This need not be the case—this must not continue to be the case. We feel persuaded that we shall have a change for the better, before we shall witness the removal of intemperance, and the renovation of the world. We are persuaded that plans will be devised and executed, for the diffusion of truth, which have not yet been attempted, nay, even thought of; that efforts and sacrifices will be made on so gigantic a scale, as to throw the puny doings of the present day completely into the shade. We are laying ourselves open to the rebuke of the apostle, of all seeking their own; not the things which are Christ's. In reference to himself and the early Christians generally, he could say, "none of us liveth to himself—but unto the Lord." He was the great centre where all their lives met. So it is now, where the great principles of the Gospel have taken full possession of the heart. Selfishness is a wretched principle, which, in the devoted Christian's heart, is daily losing ground, giving way to the hallowed influence of love to God, and to our fellow-man, which is expanding his heart wider and wider, and making the wants of the world his

* Of the nine millions annually paid by consumers of tea, £3,500,000 are paid to the crown for duty, or more than 100 per cent. About 54,000,000 of lbs. are annually exported from Canton to all parts of the world, and it is a remarkable fact that of this quantity Great Britain and Ireland alone consume nearly 32,000,000 of lbs.—being about 10,000,000 lbs. more than all the world besides.

† The average consumption of coffee in the United Kingdom is one pound per head, but in the United States it is about six pounds per head. The reasons of this difference probably are—teetotalism has spread much more extensively among them; besides which they have no duty to pay on this article. The consumption in the United States in 1841, for a population of 17,000,000, was 109,200,247 lbs.; and in the United Kingdom for the same period, for a population of 28,000,000, 28,421,466 lbs.

‡ We spend, as a nation, about £5,000,000 annually upon tobacco, about £10,000 of which goes daily to the government; and we spend £500,000 for the purpose of diffusing that truth which we believe to be essential to men's happiness in time and in eternity. What an anomaly! **Will unbelievers give us credit for sincerity? How can they?**

own; while the mass of misery arising from intemperance and sin, is constantly presenting opportunities for the employment of his utmost capabilities. He now finds that self-denial is a golden mine, containing abundance of ore—but to possess it he must dig—he must go beneath the surface—he must descend into the depths. This self-denial not only respects subduing all that is sinful, but includes abstinence even from lawful things, if thereby we can do good. That is the greatest self-denial where there is the greatest inclination, and yet such a love to Christ and our fellow-men, as excites us not only to curb or suppress it, but continually and vigorously to oppose it till conquered. This was the influence which induced Paul to say, "If meat make my brother to offend, I will not eat flesh while the world standeth." Christ laid it down as one of the fundamental laws of his kingdom, "Whosoever will come after me, let him deny himself and take up his cross, and follow me." So that we see, both in entering upon, and proceeding in the divine life, self-denial is one of its essentials. Among many other practical exhibitions of this heaven-born principle, we have pleasure in recording the following. The venerable W. Jay, says he was one day attending a missionary tea meeting, and before the close of it, a minister rose up and said he had to present a donation. The offering was not large in itself—but it showed a nobleness of disposition, and was beyond the two mites of the applauded widow. "These two guineas," said he, "are sent from a servant, who was allowed so much by her mistress for tea, but who had, during two years, denied herself the use of this beverage to aid your collection!

The sum of £6 14*s.* 4*d.* was lately presented, as sacrifice money, at a Wesleyan missionary breakfast, with a paper stating that if the 337,598 members of that society in Great Britain, would do the same, it would amount to more than £1,000,000 per annum.

This great principle is not only taught us by Scripture and Christianity—but is also the grand law of nature, inscribed by the hand of God on every part of creation. Not for itself, says the excellent Payson, but for others, does the sun disperse his beams. Not for herself but for others, does the earth unlock her treasures. Not for themselves but for others, do the clouds distill their showers. Not for themselves but for others, do the trees produce their fruits, or the flowers diffuse their fragrance and display their various hues. So, not for himself but for others, are the blessings of God bestowed upon man; and whenever, instead of diffusing them around, he devotes them exclusively to his own gratification, and shuts himself up in the dark, dreary, and flinty caverns of selfishness, he transgresseth the great law of creation—he cuts himself off from the created universe and its Author—he sacrilegiously converts to his own use, the favors which were given him for the benefit of others—and must be considered not only as unprofitable, but as a fraudulent servant who has worse than wasted his lord's money. He who thus lives to himself, and consumes the bounties of Heaven upon his lusts, or consecrates them to the demon of avarice, is a barren rock in a fertile plain—he is a thorny bramble in a fruitful vineyard—he is the very Arabia desert in the moral world. And if he is highly exalted in wealth and power, he stands inaccessible and strong, like an isolated, towering cliff, which exhibits only a cold and cheerless prospect—intercepts the genial beams of the sun—chills the vale below with its gloomy shade—adds fresh keenness to the freezing blast—and tempts down the lightning of angry Heaven. How different this from the gently rising hill, clothed to its summit with fruits and flowers, which attracts and receives the dew of heaven; and retaining only sufficient to maintain its fertility, sends down the remainder in a thousand streams, to bless the vales which lie at its feet.

After all, this self-denial is not so difficult of performance, or so unpleasant as some imagine, if a man be but influenced by heaven-born principles, and remembers that he is "created anew in Christ Jesus unto good works, which God hath before ordained that we should walk in them." Though it may involve the loss of some worldly gratification, he enjoys "the luxury of doing good"—of being doubly blessed, i. e., of being blessed, and made a blessing.

The nervous language of a late popular author is so much in point, that we cannot resist the desire of giving our readers the advantage of perusing it. He says, "Man has various appetites and desires in common with inferior animals, which are to be denied, not exterminated; to be renounced as masters, guides, or lords; and to be brought into strict and entire subordination to our moral and intellectual powers. The reason for this is, because they do not carry with them their own rule. They are blind impulses. Present their objects, and they are excited as easily when gratification would be injurious, as when it would be useless. Our desires are undiscerning instincts, generally directed to what is useful, but often clamoring for gratifications which would be injurious to health, would debilitate the mind, and oppose the general good. This blindness of desire makes the demand for self-denial urgent and continual. But besides this, when once we yield the reins to appetite, we know not where it will take us, as it always carries with it a principle of growth. It expands by indulgence, and if not restrained may prove awfully destructive. God has set bounds to the desires of the brute, but not to those of man; in brutes, for example, the animal appetites impel to a certain round of simple gratifications, beyond which they never pass. But man, having imaginations and inventions, is able by these noble faculties to whet his sensual desires to any extent. He is able to form new combinations of animal pleasures, and to provoke appetite by stimulants. The east gives up its spices, and the south holds not back its vintage; sea and land are rifled for luxuries; while the animal finds its nourishment in a few plants, perhaps in a single blade, man's table groans under the spoils of all regions;* and the consequence is, in not a few instances,

* Swift has jocosely observed, "Such is the extent of modern epicurism, that the world must be compassed before a washer-woman can sit down to breakfast," by a voyage to the east for tea and to the west for sugar.

the whole strength of the soul runs into appetite, just as some rich soil shoots up into poisonous weeds, and man, the rational creature of God, degenerates into the most thorough sensualist."

And though some may ridicule the idea, and try to laugh to scorn the man who chooses to tread this path of self-denial, yet it will be found in the end, that the history of such will most interest and absorb a discerning public. In reading the history of individuals, who is the man whom you select as the object of your special admiration? Is it he who lived to indulge himself? Whose table was most luxuriously spread? Whose current of life flowed most equally and pleasantly? Were such the men to whom monuments have been reared, and whose memories, freshened with the tears of joy and reverence, grow and flourish, and spread through every age? Oh no! It is he who has denied himself; who has made the most entire sacrifice of appetite and private interest to God and mankind; who has walked in a rugged path, and clung to good and great ends, in persecution and pain; who, amidst the solicitations of ambition, ease, and private friendship, and the menaces of tyranny and malice, has listened to the voice of conscience, and found a recompense for blighted hopes and protracted sufferings in conscious uprightness, and the favor of God.

Who is most lovely in domestic life? It is the martyr to domestic affliction; the mother forgetting herself, and ready to suffer, toil, and die for the happiness of her children. Who is it that we honor most in public life? It is the martyr to his country; he who serves her, not when she has honors for his brow, and wealth for his coffers, but who clings to her in her dangers and falling glories, and thinks life a cheap sacrifice to her safety and freedom. Whom does the church retain in most grateful remembrance? The self-denying apostle, the fearless confessor, the devoted martyr; men who have held fast the truth even in death, and bequeathed it to future ages amidst blood. Above all, to what moment of the life of Christ does the Christian turn, as the most affecting and sublime illustration of his divine charity? It is the moment when, in the spirit of self-denial, he bore the agony and shame of the cross.

"Thus all great virtues bear the impress of self-denial; and were God's present constitution of our nature and life so reversed, as to demand no renunciation of desire, the chief interest and glory of our present being would pass away. There would be nothing in history to thrill us with admiration. We should have no consciousness of the power and greatness of the soul. We should love feebly and coldly, for we should find nothing in one another to love earnestly."

Let us not then complain that Providence has made self-denial necessary, or that the blessed Jesus has made it a chief ingredient in his religion, and thus summons us to the work; it is for our interest. Organic and moral law here hold one language, and our own souls bear witness to the teaching of Christ, that while it is eminently calculated to promote our health of body, it is also the "narrow way which leadeth unto life." Thus self-denial "hath the promise of the life that now is, and of that which is to come." The practice of self-denial will also have an important bearing on our dying circumstances. If at that moment our reason is spared to us, and memory retains its hold on the past, will it gratify us to see that we have lived, not to deny, but to indulge ourselves? That we have bound our souls to any passions? That we gave the reins to lust; that we were palsied by sloth; that through the love of gain we hardened ourselves against the claims of humanity; or through the love of man's favor we parted with truth and moral independence; or that in any thing reason and conscience were sacrificed to the impulse of desire, and God forgotten for present good? Shall we then find comfort in remembering our tables of luxury, our pillows of down, our wealth amassed and employed for private ends, or our honors won by base compliance with the world? Did any man, in his dying moments, ever regret his conflicts with himself—his victories over appetite—his scorn of impure pleasures—or his sufferings in a righteous cause? Did any man ever mourn that he had impoverished himself in the service of mankind? Are these the recollections which harrow up the soul, and darken and appall the last hour? To whom is the last hour most serene and full of hope? Is it not to him, who, amidst perils and allurements has denied himself, taken up his cross, and followed the self-denying Jesus?

Thus you see, to deny ourselves is to withstand, to renounce whatever without or within interferes with our convictions of right, with the claims of mankind, our conscience, and our God. It is to suffer, to make sacrifices for our principles. The conduct of Jesus is our guide. He not only came to teach us religion, but also to show it forth in himself, to personify it. He is not a mere channel through which certain communications are made to flow from God; not a mere messenger, appointed to utter the words which he had heard, and then to disappear, and to sustain no further connection with his message. He came to be a living manifestation of his religion. This is a peculiarity worthy of attention, showing that Christianity is not a mere code of laws—not an abstract system, but a living, embodied religion. It comes to us in a human form; it offers itself to our eyes as well as our ears; it breathes, it moves in our sight; it is more than precept, it is example and action.

Let our readers, if they lay claim to the Christian character, hasten to conform themselves to Christ, and to the laws of his kingdom; in doing which they will promote the glory of "God in the highest, peace on earth, and good-will among men;" they will reap the advantage of it in their own souls. "Millions yet unborn will call them blessed, and when they have run the race of life, their dying moments will be cheered by the pleasing recollection, that they have labored to promote the good" of the world.

APPENDIX.

Temperance Orders—(A.) Page 17.

Seven years ago, temperance beneficial societies were first instituted in the United States. The most prominent order existing is that of the Sons of Temperance. This order now comprises a National Division, thirty-five Grand Divisions, about five thousand subordinate Divisions, with two hundred and fifty thousand contributing members. Besides this moral army of permanently organized teetotalers, there are various other associations adopting the total abstinence and mutual assurance basis, the principal of which are the Rechabites, the Temples of Honor, the Cadets of Temperance, and the Daughters of Temperance. Add to these the Washingtonians and other total abstainers, unconnected with any particular organization, and we have a million pledged foes to King Alcohol, nearly all recruited within the last quarter of a century.

Excessive Stimulation—(B.) Page 24.

That excessive stimulation—all artificial stimulation is excessive—not only wears out the vital organism prematurely, but throws the machinery of life into disorder, whereby deaths occur suddenly and violently, is proved by every day's experience in civilized society. Our witnesses are fevers, inflammations, convulsions, cholera, consumption, etc. The most deplorable aspect in which we can view the effects of a hurried and disorderly working of the organic functions is that of hereditary transmission. The offspring of the parent who transgresses the laws of life and health are frequently the greatest, and always the most pitiful sufferers. A man born with an originally powerful constitution, may indulge in all manner of "riotous living," and endure to sixty or seventy years, while his offspring, to whom he has bequeathed his acquired infirmities, cannot hold out, under the same excesses, more than forty or fifty years. How sacred the duty, how awful the responsibility of parents, in this relation!

Distillery Milk—(C.) Page 49.

In the cities of New-York and Brooklyn, and in the village of Williamsburg, many thousands of cows are kept in close, ill-ventilated, and horribly filthy stables, fed on distillery slops, and every other kind of foul, refuse material; and their milk, which is an absolute poison, is sold to our citizens, and swallowed by our infantile population. The animals thus treated soon become diseased, when they are killed, and their carcasses peddled out to the people, under the name of beef. Although books have been written on this subject, and although the press has, during the last ten years, often and repeatedly called the attention of the sovereign people and the constituted authorities to these enormous evils, they still remain unchecked and untouched. The rights of property appear to have a much stronger claim on legislating powers than the rights of persons. The right of a rich man to get richer, in the prosecution of a nuisance-business, is regarded higher than the right of a poor man to live! Because "private rights," as the phrase goes, are not to be meddled with; the public, who happen to be too ignorant to know their wrongs, or too feeble to defend their rights, may be cheated, defrauded, maimed, robbed, and poisoned, all because a certain select, few, privileged, rich distillers find it profitable to sell their putrescent slops to be manufactured into a fluid resembling milk, after having converted the natural food of man—the grains and fruits which God gave him to eat—into alcoholic poison. If there is a business on earth pre-eminently nefarious, it is this; if there is any system of legislation more thoroughly barbarian than all others, it is that which cherishes and protects the property principle at the expense of the image of God!

Moderate Drinkers—(D.) Page 59.

These "devil's decoys" are the greatest obstacles in the way of all reforms. The man who deals in intoxicating liquors in a palace, and preserves the external forms of respectability, has an influence for evil which the low grog-shop keeper, the loafer, can make no pretensions to. So with the moderate drinker. He maintains a respectable exterior; his position in society is honorable; he "can drink or let it alone." His counsel is listened to, and his example followed by others. Not so with the gutter-drunkard, or the immoderate drinker. No one considers his condition or ways exemplary. He rather serves as a frightful example to warn others from treading in his footsteps; while the man of character and station misleads others into his downward habits, many of whom inevitably become miserable and ruined drunkards. When I hear of a learned professor, an eminent statesman, a distinguished physician, or a Christian minister, who advocates or practices the moderate use of wine, I am always reminded of the devil's decoy.

Diet at Graefenburg—(E.) Page 66.

Much has been said and written about the unphysiological character of a portion of the dietary system at Priessnitz's establishment. Persons not accustomed to provide a table for water-cure patients, can have little idea of the difficulty of controlling artificial appetites. Imagine a man surrounded by five hundred invalids, all having their opinions, conceits, and prejudices; all having been long addicted to improper or intemperate eating and drinking; all full of morbid cravings, and, in exact ratio to their intensity, incapable of self-control; most of them, too, nervous, peevish, irritable, and fault-finding, because the consequences of over-indulgence demand self-denial and privation as indispensable conditions of restoration; and some conception may be formed of the herculean task of carrying out any dietetic arrangement on strictly physiological rules. It is true that some articles of food, usually found on the table at Graefenburg, are positively bad; and the greater part of the dietary system would admit of improvement. It is not to be supposed that Priessnitz, with all his vastness and originality of mind, has had the opportunity of investigating theoretically and reducing to practice all the details of a physiological regimen. To his great credit, however, and evincive of his quick perception and accurate observation, be it said, that his special directions to his patients as to what food is best for them, are singularly judicious and philosophical, according with the more profound investigations of Graham, Lambe, and other dietetic reformers. He gives them to understand, in general terms, that the more simple and plain their food the sooner they may expect to recover health. He tells them that coarse, unconcentrated food is the best, eaten cool or cold; that brown or unbolted meal is far preferable to fine or superfine for the farinaceous part of their diet; he teaches them that the most rapid and perfect cures are made by abandoning all animal food; that simple brown bread and pure water are sufficient in themselves for perfect nutrition, and then leaves them to their own responsibility. What more could one man do among so many, whose appetites were ten times as strong as their wills? Although he did not, amid the opposition and persecution which surrounded and embarrassed him, strictly carry out his own views of diet, he has taken a position far in advance of the medical profession, and which, fifty years hence, like the writings of Graham, Lambe, Alcott, Smith, and Cornaro, will be better understood and appreciated than now.

Animal Fat—(F.) Page 69.

Nothing more strongly illustrates the utter absurdity and total want of all philosophical principle, in the popular medical practice of the day, than this plan of relieving particular symptoms at the expense of the general health. This applies to the dietetic as well as the medicinal treatment. Heartburn indicates acidity, foul secretion, morbid matter in the stomach, or decomposed, unhealthy, and acrid bile in the *duodenum*, near the lower orifice of the stomach. It is so much easier to quiet this feeling for the time than to cure it permanently, that the doctors generally content themselves with smothering the sensation, while they allow the causes to go on undisturbed. They *tinker* away at the effect without thinking of the condition. Almost any stimulating substance, as brandy, pepper, mustard; or alkaline material, as soda, magnesia, saleratus; or greasy compound, as fat pork, bacon, cod liver oil, will allay or overcome the feeling for a time. But this is only stifling the outcries of nature, and changing the form of disease into less apparent, but really more destructive conditions. Medical books are full of inconsistencies in theory and contradictions in experience on the subject of greasy foods, fat meats, and animal oils.

Liebig imagines that fat, employed as food, serves an important part in the animal economy, by supplying carbon to be "burnt in the lungs," thus supporting respiration and promoting animal heat. He has entirely and most strangely overlooked the obvious fact, that the offensive carbon is merely thrown off in this way; got rid of as useless and effete matter

This chemical theory of Liebig, which makes fat an alimentary principle, also makes alcohol an alimentary principle. Alcohol is a highly noxious, and highly carbonated liquid. The organism resents, rejects, and expels it in all possible ways. Much of its plus-carbon is ejected from the lungs by means of the respiratory function. The increased chemical and physiological action requisite to get rid of it, of course increases the animal heat temporarily; but so far from this process, this preternatural augmentation of heat, being a useful way to support respiration, it is an absolute febrile and injurious effect, tending to exhaust the vitality, and prematurely wear out the organic machinery.

Now, strange as it may seem, Pereira, in his able work on food and diet—able in the chemical sense only, does actually, on the ground I am controverting, declare alcohol an alimentary principle! I only wonder that, following out this wild vagary, tobacco was not made an alimentary principle. "The filthy weed" is in very general use; it contains much carbon; and one has only to smell the breath of a tobacco-eater to discover that some of its elements are expelled from the system through the lungs. Why not then say, tobacco furnishes carbon to be "burnt in the lungs," thus supporting respiration, thus maintaining the animal heat, and thus becoming an important alimentary principle! Ridiculous as is this conclusion, it results legitimately from the premises assumed in relation to the uses of animal oils. Such are the egregious errors resulting from the substitution of mere chemical analyses, always imperfect, for physiological principles, always true and immutable.

Pereira says: "Fixed oil or fat is more difficult of digestion, and more obnoxious to the stomach, than any other alimentary principle." Is not this good ground to suspect it is not an alimentary principle at all? Surely nature cannot be so inconsistent as to provide an indigestible and obnoxious alimentary principle! But, *per contra,* Professor C. A. Lee, of this city, in editing Pereira's work, tells us that he has treated many cases of cholera infantum, where every thing would be rejected from the stomach except salt pork, or fat bacon, rare broiled, and given in small quantities at a time. Here is another delusion of theory. Because a given article of food, or medicine, or poison, will resist the efforts of the stomach to expel it, when the digestive organs are incapable of acting on any nutritive material, and when no food at all should be forced into the stomach, it by no means follows that such article is best. When the stomach rejects particular articles of medicine, the physician is very apt to try one drug after another, until something stays on the stomach. Then he imagines that he has achieved a great victory. Perhaps he has; and conquered the stomach instead of the disease. The allopathic system is mainly practiced on the principle of silencing the efforts of nature. It is a mischievous practice, whether in the use of calomel and opium as remedies, or fat pork and bacon as victuals.

How much more rational and common-sensical is it, in cholera cases, as instanced by Dr. Lee, to give the patient plenty of tepid or cool water to dilute and wash away the offending material in the stomach, then let it alone until rest and restoration allow the *natural appetite* to determine when food is wanted and can be digested.

THEORY OF STIMULATION—(G.) Page 71.

The common notions of stimulation entertained by the medical faculty, have led to a practice incalculably injurious. When the digestive organs have been worn down, as it were, with excitement, over-burdened with concentrated and improper aliment, and over-worked by stimulating food, drinks, nervines, condiments, etc., it is the general practice to undertake to counteract the consequences by giving additional intensity to the causes; that is, to lash up the stomach, digestive powers, and nervous system to additional efforts by new, and ever-varied, and constantly increasing stimulants. This is exactly analogous to whipping a horse whose strength has been overtasked by too heavy a load. The application of the lash causes the abused animal to expend his vitality faster than he could in any natural use of his muscles, and he *seems* stronger. But nobody supposes a horse thus treated will live as long or do as much work during his natural life as one whose exhausted strength was invigorated by rest instead of violence.

To re-invigorate the exhausted digestive powers of the human animal, rest and quiet are nature's indications. This implies the absence of all stimulating or irritating ingesta. We know that in a depressed state of the vital powers, in those accustomed to various stimuli, stimulating food *feels* the most agreeable for the moment; and in these cases animal food, to those in the habit of using it, of course, feels more pleasant than vegetable. But it oppresses the body more in the end by its very power of stimulation. I have treated many bad cases of dyspepsia, and my experience has been uniformly and most decidedly in favor of the *strictest* vegetable diet. The great advantage of this consists, in my opinion, in its greater purity of material, in its natural adaptation to the human constitution, and in its complete destitution of all stimulating properties.

Animal Fat in Cold Climates—(H.) Page 71.

This "best reason" will appear one of the very worst when rightly apprehended. The fact that people *can bear* in a very cold climate what would kill them outright in a very warm one, does not prove that they can do no better. Persons in temperate latitudes can bear, in the winter season, a kind and degree of gross, greasy, and impure animal food, which, in the summer season, would immediately endanger their lives. For what other reason are oysters adjudged, by popular sentiment, to be unhealthy during the months which have no letter *r*—the four hottest months of the year? The only scientific argument yet brought to bear in favor of animal fat, or animal food, in a cold climate, is the carbonic theory of respiration. This I have attended to in the preceding note. I will further remark in this place, that the carbonaceous theorists singularly enough seem to overlook the fact, that the various kinds of vegetable food known, contain as much carbon as the various kinds of animal food in use. Nature has not done her work so blunderingly as to forget to put the proper quantity of carbon in the purest and best kinds of food. It is true that the fixed oils, both animal and vegetable, contain a much larger quantity of carbon than other forms of animal and vegetable matters do. But ample experience has demonstrated that all oily matters are the very poorest dietetic substances, even if they are useful at all. In every part of the earth, the people whose diet consists of a large proportion of animal oils, are among the lowest and most degraded of the human family, physically and mentally. Those who refer to the diminutive and deformed Esquimaux, who devour immense quantities of train oil, as evidence of the necessity or utility of fat in a cold climate, should be reminded of the Russian Cossacks, and a tribe of Finlanders, who inhabit an extremely rigorous latitude, subsisting on the most simple and rather scanty vegetable fare, and who enjoy a high degree of physical strength, symmetry, and activity.

It has long been a popular fallacy that alcohol was necessary in cold climates; but recently Sir John Ross and other North-sea navigators have dispelled this delusion by actual experiment. Similar experiments, I have no manner of doubt, would dispel the similar error in relation to blubber oil and fat meats.

Digestibility of Food—(I.) Page 73.

The capacity of the stomach to digest any given article of food is so much a matter of habit, that no correct conclusions can be drawn from the first effect of any kind the stomach has not been accustomed to. The digestive powers are also very much modified by the sum total of all our voluntary habits. Persons who have been for a considerable time trained to a correct vegetable regimen, can eat, not only with impunity, but with pleasure and profit, cabbage, cucumbers, spinage, asparagus, simply boiled, and even many esculent roots without any preparation at all; whereas, in a stomach just from its concentrated food, stimulating flesh, warming condiments, and enervating hot drinks, they might produce a regular fit of colic. The same remarks apply to various kinds of nuts, which in some produce extreme indigestion, while others can use them with entire impunity. The fallacy of reasoning from the immediate feeling produced in the stomach depraved by false ingesta, thus taking a morbid habit to guide us instead of an ascertained physiological principle, may be well illustrated by referring to the article of old cheese. What is called old, rich, strong cheese, is, in my judgment, one of the most indigestible, injurious, I had almost said *poisonous*, articles of diet known. Yet it is in extensive use; and most persons say it feels well in the stomach. Indeed, many persons who eat pretty heavy dinners take a piece of it as a "digester," just as others do a glass of brandy. That it is essentially a bad thing I have proved in the following manner—I have known several persons who have disused it several months, living at the same time on plain food, mostly vegetable. In this way the natural sensibility of the tongue, palate, throat, stomach, etc., was measurably restored. On eating a moderately sized piece of good, old, rich cheese, a "canker in the mouth," and a constipated state of the bowels would always exist the next day. I have known the experiment repeated, and have tried it several times myself, always with these results.

Theory of Population—(J.) Page 78.

The doctrine of "divine permission," as commonly understood and applied to our voluntary habits, has been productive of much confusion in theology, as it has of mischief in hygiene. Regarding God as the great first cause, we must, of necessity, admit that nothing can happen without his permission. But to suppose that animal food and alcoholic liquors were permitted man to shorten his life, and prevent an excessive growth of wickedness, according to Dr. Cheyne, is indirectly charging the Almighty with at least a very cruel and awkward way of accomplishing a desirable end. More consistent is it with his attributes, and more consonant with a rational philosophy, to suppose that he permits us to infringe his laws, that he gives us ability to act, in our very limited sphere, against the general order of nature, for the benevolent purpose of teaching us that order. This, it may be presumed, can be done in no better way than by making us practically acquainted with the blessings of conforming our lives to his laws, and the miseries inseparably connected with their infraction. Good and evil, in this sense, may be said to be "permitted," and intended to teach us, by our own individual experience, the relations of cause and effect; in other words, the laws by which we, and all the universe of matter and of mind, are, have been, and ever will be governed.

Philosophers have been much puzzled in their attempts to make out a satisfactory theory of population. Mr. Malthus has contended that population has a tendency to increase faster than the means of subsistence, unless some extraordinary counteracting causes be interposed. On this assumption, "war, pestilence, and famine" may be hailed as special godsends, to keep the race down to the level of the means of subsistence; but it places the Creator in an attitude from which our reason revolts. Mr. Doubleday, on the other hand, has lately met the positions of Mr. Malthus with an opposite theory. He has undertaken to show that poverty is the great cause of a rapid increase, and that a good degree of the comforts of life "deadens the principle of increase." He proves the first clause of his proposition by adverting to the fact that poor folks have the most children; and the latter part by quoting the well-known historical data, that wealthy and luxurious families very frequently run out, as have done wealthy and luxurious nations. The doctrines of both these gentlemen are too narrow and superficial to be worthy of God, or honorable to man. They are both mistaken, I think, in endeavoring to turn man's abuse of natural laws into "natural tendencies."

Great wealth and extreme poverty are equally in violation of the "natural constitution of man." That God who made the earth, fashioned it to produce sustenance enough for all the beings created in his own image. If men have got at variance with themselves, warred upon each other; if some have usurped too much of the domain of our common mother earth, and others have not where to lay their heads; if men have deranged their proper social relations, perverted the laws of their own organization, and entailed upon themselves and society innumerable "permitted" evils, let them pause long before they charge all these results to "natural tendencies." When men live according to the laws of their being, extreme wealth and extreme poverty, by which one portion of mankind are pampered to death and the other starved, will soon cease to exist; and there will be no more trouble about either excessive or deficient population. Look over the world. In some of the European nations, it takes the labor of a hundred or a thousand peasants, or serfs, to maintain one young sprig of nobility in a life of fashionable dissipation. In nearly all countries, a vast amount of toil and talent is wasted in miscultivating the earth for tobacco, coffee, tea, and other injurious narcotics and nervines; and an immense amount of the natural food of the human family, grains and fruits, is manufactured into alcoholic poisons. So long as man ravages the earth instead of ruling it, so long as he plays tyrant instead of lord over it, and over the rest of the animal creation, so long will the theory of population be an unsolved problem, to those who cannot distinguish between man's transgressions and God's designs.

Much has been said about the Mosaic regulations concerning diet, etc. Moses was, no doubt, a sagacious legislator, and a much better physiologist than most doctors now-a-days who undertake to direct the eating habits of the people. He had, it must be recollected, an ignorant, sensual, semi-barbarous people to deal with, such as are a majority of the human race at this day. His teachings in relation to their personal habits were as much "in advance of the age" as he could have had any reasonable expectation they could appreciate, or would practice Hence his permission to eat the very best kinds of animal food, so long as he could not at once raise their depraved appetites above the flesh-pots which "their souls lusted after," while he gave specific directions to lead them into the ways of personal cleanliness, bodily purity, and better health, shows him to have been a philosopher of the progressive school.

Let the reformer of the present day, be he theological or physiological, set up a standard of moral life, or a law of eating and drinking, in all respects strictly adapted to the laws of God and nature, and the best condition and highest happiness of the whole human family, and how many could he induce to "walk therein?" We should all be Moses-like, and try to lead erring humanity to truth and nature, step by step, always keeping the standard of reform as far in advance of the mass of the people as they can distinctly perceive and be induced to follow.

Is Man a Drinking Animal?—(K.) Page 95.

This is a disputed point. Dr. Lambe, of London, has argued very ably that man is not naturally a drinking animal. The great majority of dietetic writers hold the opposite opinion, while a few think his best condition requires him to drink largely, even at meals. There can be no doubt—indeed, Dr. Alcott and others have proved it by direct experiment—that those who adopt a vegetable regimen and make a large proportion of their food consist of succulent fruits and watery vegetables, can be perfectly sustained and nourished without water-drinking. It is also certain that those who employ greasy dishes, who eat much animal food, and who use salt and spices freely, or who partake freely of concentrated farinaceous preparations, find a large quantity of water, as drink, necessary to carry off the saline particles and other impurities, and assuage the factitious fever of the organism. This, though, is not nature, but a perversion of it. I think in all cases the thirst is the safe rule to go by. All persons should be sure and have *pure* fresh water. Hard water ought certainly never to be used as a drink, or for culinary purposes. I am convinced that the habit of drinking much at meals is wrong, unless, as I have just remarked, thirst is provoked by stimulating food, condiments, or seasonings.

Stimulating Water—(L.) Page 99.

Richerand's expression—"The purest water is rendered stimulating by the air and salts it contains," is one of those unaccountable absurdities which have, in some strange way, got into the heads and books of a large class of men calling themselves scientific. Pure water is entirely free from all saline ingredients; and is not in the least degree stimulating. It is simply nutritious and solvent. It enters largely into all the solid structures of the body, forms the greater part of the fluids, serves as a vehicle to carry the elements of reparation and growth to all parts of the system, and the effete, or waste particles, from the organism through the several excretions. This view of its uses shows at once why it should not be in any sense or degree saline nor stimulating. Waters which contain various salts, earthy matters, alkalies, or mineral substances, like our famous Spas, are fruitful sources of disease. The great number of medicinal springs, so celebrated in all parts of the fashionable world, for curing the fashionable complaints of fashionable folks, owe their whole fame to the ridiculous fashionable conceit, that impure water, which is not fit for healthy people to swallow, is much the healthiest for fashionably sick persons.

Alcoholic Medicines—(M.) Page 101.

The employment of alcoholic liquors, as medicines, by so large a portion of the medical faculty, is, in my opinion, the greatest stumbling-block in the way of the temperance reformation. So long as the various forms of intoxicating drinks are used as remedies, they will be abused as beverages; and so long will innumerable quacks drive a flourishing trade in selling sweetened liquors, moderately drugged, under the names of Sarsaparilla Extracts, Life Balsams, Purifying Syrups, Anti-dyspeptic Bitters, Anti-bilious Cordials, etc., etc. The *regular* trade may thank their own bad example for such a prosperous state of the business of their rivals of the *irregular* trade.

Several eminent medical men—as eminent as any among the living or dead—have expressed their decided conviction that all alcoholic medicines were, to say the least, unnecessary. They have given, too, many weighty reasons for such a conclusion; yet, although I am not aware of a sound argument in their favor ever being advanced, their routine and most empyrical employment continues almost unabated in force to this moment. It is not a little singular that so many homœopathic practitioners, who profess to administer the materia medica on a principle totally opposite to the doctrine of the allopathists, give the alcoholic stimulants generally in allopathic quantities.

It is perhaps impossible to make physicians or people comprehend, so long as all the poisons of the mineral, vegetable, and animal kingdoms are recognized by the faculty as remedies, why the alcoholic poison should not be in the catalogue. We see, therefore, but little encouragement without directing the battering-rams of temperance reform against the apothecary shop.

To clear the authorized pharmacopœia of its "ardent spirits, malt liquors, wine, and cider," we shall probably be obliged to annihilate the whole tribe of drugs and destructives, an achievement, by the way, which, when accomplished, will do more to preserve the public health than all the sanatory statutes enacted since the world began.

I cannot here refrain from administering a little reproof to a certain class of temperance men, on the subject of practical total abstinence; I mean those who have pledged themselves not to drink the alcoholic bane, but who continue to *eat* it. It is an every-day affair for such persons to cry aloud, "plum-pudding—wine," at the refectories; to eat brandied steaks, brandied mince-pies, and brandied sweet-meats, or cakes and gravies in which wine constitutes one of the component parts. Thus they observe the mere letter of the pledge and trample on its spirit. This is a pitiful exhibition of pretended philanthropy; and the man must be grossly the slave of a perverted appetite, or lamentably blind in his understanding of the temperance principle, or sadly deficient in the spirit of true humanity, who can, for a moment's gratification of a morbid taste, commend to his fellow-creatures the eating principle of alcoholic stimulation, while peradventure he is in the habit of declaiming often, long, loud, and strong against its drinking practice.

Salt—(N.) Page 102.

Probably no article, as a mere condiment or seasoning, is less harmful than salt, if used very moderately. But I am fully persuaded its ordinary free use is highly injurious. As a dietetic article I regard it as worse than useless—common opinion, and the frequent assertions of medical books to the contrary notwithstanding. The free use of salt irritates the mouth, throat, and stomach, creating thirst and fever, and provoking unnatural appetite, while it loads the circulating fluids with a foreign ingredient, which the excretory organs must labor inordinately to get rid of. It produces glandular obstructions, rigidity of fibre, stiffness of muscles, and impoverished blood. The antiseptic quality of salt has been often alleged as a ground of its utility; but this is precisely the quality that renders it most unfit for nutritive purposes. Perfect digestion requires the most easy transformation of the alimentary materials—not easy in point of time, but in respect to purity and congeniality of proximate elements. The antiseptic quality of salt renders the alimentary substances with which it mixes and combines, particularly the fibrous portion of animal food, hard, insoluble, and so far indigestible. That well-known putrescent condition of the body, called scurvy, so common among sailors confined for a long time to salted provisions, is at least strong presumptive evidence against its utility. On chemical grounds, it is argued that most of the vegetable and animal substances employed as food, contain a greater or less proportion of the elements of common salt—soda and hydro-chloric acid. To this it is a sufficient reply, that nature has put the elements of our food together in exactly the right proportion, those substances containing precisely what the organic economy requires, so that we need make no extraneous additions.

Causes of Cholera—(O.) Page 117.

The prevalence of cholera during the past season, has caused an immense amount of crimination, unmeaning, of course, to be uttered against the Most High, from high places and low places. Nothing is more common than to hear this pestilence spoken of as the "scourge of the Almighty," the "mysterious dealings of Providence," the "wrath of the Deity," etc., etc. It seems to be much easier to blaspheme God and libel nature than to mend our own manners when evils beset us. "Fasting, humiliation, and prayer" are all commendable, when intelligently exercised; but when, in view of any prevailing epidemic disease, we pray God to "avert His anger," while we continue to practice our own misdeeds, which are in fact the causes of the epidemic, our devotion can have no moral character above that of solemn mockery. His will, and His power, to "stay the pestilence," will always be coupled with the condition, that we cease to transgress the laws of our being. It is an historical truth that, in all parts of the world, so far as we can derive any authentic data, no person whose voluntary habits were physiologically correct, has died of this disease. In this city we can find no account of any person who lived on plain, unconcentrated vegetable food, and fruits of good quality, and drank nothing but pure water, having ever died of cholera; nor do I believe such a case will ever be known. This is true of 1832, 1834, and 1849—all the years it has visited us. I know the contrary has been often asserted, and is perhaps generally believed, and I know, too, that the assertion is wholly false.

I can imagine no disease more artificially induced, more clearly the result of the false customs of society, more evidently the consequence of our own voluntary habits than the Asiatic cholera; and what is true of people in one part of the world is true of all. Whatever may be the remote or exciting causes of this disease, or any disease, it is very clear to my own mind that we can never have *the* cholera unless a morbid condition exists within ourselves, upon which those remote and exciting causes operate; and this condition, being the aggregate result of all our habits of life, is perfectly within our own control.

HIGH CHARGES—(P.) Page 121.

On this subject, as on all others, we should examine both sides. It is very true that hydropathic establishments *might* be so arranged and managed as to be able to treat patients at one half, or less, the usual rates. It would require, however, more capital and patronage than hydropaths have thus far enjoyed. In this country, an establishment must be got up with considerable attention to comfort and appearances, or it will not be patronized at all. It is much more expensive to keep a good establishment than a common boarding-house, as any one can understand by looking at the machinery, attendants, wear and tear, etc., required. Moreover, there are always frequent applications from "charity patients," invalids who have expended all their substance through the kind attentions of doctors and apothecaries, and who come penniless to the water-cure as a last resort. Many of these the hydropath, if he has a few drops of the milk of human kindness in his composition, cannot turn away. He must take them, board, lodge, supply, and attend them for just what they have to pay—"be the same more or less." Now, if he graduated his scale of charges at the lowest living rates to the paying class, the non-paying, unless he hardened his heart, would inevitably sink him. It may be said that the poor *ought* to have friends who should each contribute a little to their expenses, or the public might assist them instead of the hydropath bearing all the burden. All this *might* be so; but it is not infrequently quite otherwise. If a benevolent public, or if philanthropic individuals of wealth could be induced to construct the right kind of establishments, so that system, association, and capital could be combined, the expenses could be reduced proportionately.

Drugged Liquors—(Q.) Page 124.

To the list of adulterating agents named in the text, in *common* use by the manufacturers of intoxicating drinks, may be added various essential oils, logwood, Brazil-wood, alum, green vitriol, capsicum, bitter oranges, sugar of lead, oil of bitter almonds, India berry, poke berries, elder berries, poison hemlock, laurel water, prussic acid, dragon's blood, lamb's blood, gum benzoin, red sanders, burnt sugar, salt of tartar, and many others. A late author on chemistry, enumerates *forty-six* adulterating ingredients employed in the manufacture of beer alone. Nine tenths of the sweet wines in market are extensively adulterated. In fact, the greater proportion of all the liquors of commerce consist of alcoholic poison, drugged with still other poisons.

"When Doctor's Disagree"—(R.) Page 125.

Dr. C. Herring has related the following anecdote: While traveling through Germany, he was invited to the house of a rich old gentleman, who had been an invalid for twenty years. This gentleman had at first consulted two physicians of celebrity, but as they quarreled about his complaint, he determined to seek other advice. But first he resolved, that if he could find three doctors who perfectly agreed upon his case without hesitation, to allow himself to be treated by them, but not otherwise. For this purpose he had consulted many eminent physicians, whose advice and prescriptions he had recorded in a book kept for the purpose, which, as may be supposed, had cost him a pretty sum of money, but never found any three who agreed respecting his case.

This book had the appearance of a ledger in large folio, and was kept in the form of tables. In the first column were the names of the physicians, amounting to 477; in the second, those of the disease, with explanations concerning its nature; of these there were 313, differing importantly from each other; in the third column were the remedies proposed; these consisted of 832 prescriptions, containing in all 1097 remedies. The sum total of fees appeared at the end of each page.

Progress of Hydropathy—(S.) Page 129.

In the United States, the doctrines of water-cure have progressed with a rapidity unparalleled by any other reformatory innovation on established usages. The oldest establishment in this country only dates back six years; now there are probably more than one hundred. Another evidence of the constantly increasing interest felt in this subject, is the great number of books and periodicals constantly emanating from the press on this subject. The Water-Cure Journal, published by Fowlers and Wells, in this city—the oldest and leading hydropathic periodical of this country, has attained an extent of circulation equaled by few monthlies in the world, and is now acquiring readers and patrons faster than ever before.

CUTANEOUS TRANSPIRATION—(T.) Page 142.

The experiment mentioned in the text does not prove that every person ought to expel through the skin from four and a half to five and a half pounds of effete material; but that some persons do. The quantity of perspirable matter in different individuals must vary according to their general habits of life, particularly as regards exercise, food, and drink.

That we "feed upon air," is literally true. The skin is without doubt, in some degree, a breathing organ. It is capable of absorbing a certain amount of water, thus in some measure allaying thirst; and its ability to derive nourishment of the more ethereal kind, the vital or electrical principle, from the surrounding atmosphere, is in my mind unquestionable. In this sense, however, its principal function is that of a regulator. Persons of open, porous, vigorous skins, can bear with impunity alternations of temperature and varying electrical states, which, to those whose cutaneous vessels are obstructed, torpid, feeble and inactive, would prove injurious or even fatal. Hence the importance of regular, daily, cold bathing, especially to those who spend much time in-doors, and bundle themselves up, after the manner of most people, in a surplus quantity of flannel.

Oxygen and Respiration—(U.) Page 150.

The idea that oxygen is a *heating* agent is no better grounded than the opposite opinion, sometimes advanced, that it is a *cooling* agent. The more rational view appears to be this: respiration is a process which aids powerfully in the regulation of the animal temperature. The oxygen of the atmosphere certainly performs an important part in the organic economy, such as combining with and aiding the expulsion of effete carbon, or, to use the modern chemical phrase, "burning the carbon in the lungs;" also, supplying the electrical principle to the blood, or, to speak more *modernly*, the magnetic element to the nerves. The animal machine is, to a greater extent than is generally supposed, self-regulating; a harmonious balance of all its functions gives it its best vital condition; and this will be warming or cooling, according to the necessities of the case. Free respiration calls into play many muscles, organs, and functions; this general activity and balance of the several systems which compose the one organism, appropriate what is useful from surrounding media, and reject what is injurious, thus defending the body alike from extremes of heat or cold; but it is a very partial investigation of the phenomena of life which imputes the combined results of the respiratory function to the chemical properties of oxygen alone.

Exercise and Sensible Perspiration—(V.) Page 153.

This rule for exercising will hardly do for all, without some qualifications. Those who live simply, bathe regularly, and exercise much habitually, sweat but very little under severe exertion. With them, sensible perspiration is no rule of action. The sensations of heat and fatigue are their better guides. That perspiration which is necessary to waste, change, disorganize, and re-compose, is mainly insensible. The profuse sweating so generally observed upon laborers and others, when exercising severely, is, to a great extent, the pouring out of the surplus fluid demanded by thirst-provoking habits of eating and drinking.

General Ablutions—(W.) Page 156.

For rubbing the surface of the body, and the processes of bathing or friction, coarse cloths appear to me far better than a sponge. The greater facility with which they can be handled is no small argument in their favor. I never apply any strong shock to the head, as a douche, or large, compact stream. The pouring bath, or shower, may be applied to the head moderately in persons whose circulation is not materially unbalanced. Those liable to headache after bathing, or subject to what is called a "rush of blood to the head," had better only wet the head with the hand or sponge.

Cutaneous Exhalations—(X.) Page 159.

Few persons seem to have a correct idea of the *natural smell* of a human being. It is a common and rather vulgar prejudice, that the strong, rank, fetid odor, that often exhales from the body of a laboring man in a state of perspiration, and the stench which frequently arises from the feet of a man who wears flannel stockings and uses no foot baths, indicates strength, health, and animal vigor. This mistake appears rather foolish on examination. All these persons, by adopting regular bathing habits and eating wholesome food, will soon lose the whole of this filthy and most *unnatural* smell. If the outlets of the body are clogged up with dead, putrescent particles, which ought to be expelled, and the pores of the skin are obstructed by decayed and waste *rotting* matter, which ought to be cleaned out, the sweat or steam arising from the body will necessarily be charged with offensive effluvia. To smell sweet, a human being has only to keep clean.

The Rubbing Wet Sheet—(Y.) Page 161.

The method of throwing the sheet *over* the head is very awkward, and entirely unnecessary. Wrapping it closely around the neck, enveloping all the body except the head, is much more convenient, and equally useful. This is one of the best of the water-cure appliances; and competent of itself, if perseveringly employed, in conjunction with a proper regimen, to cure many chronic diseases.

The Wet Sheet Pack—(Z.) Page 162.

The wet sheet packing process admits of the exercise of considerable tact and dexterity on the part of the attendant. Patients often speak of comfortable or disagreeable sensations, as they are packed skillfully or bunglingly. The head should be raised on pillows sufficiently to rest perfectly at ease. The blankets or comfortables should be spread next to the mattrass, so that the body can be enveloped more evenly and rapidly. Care should be taken to fold the clothing closely about the neck, yet not so as to be oppressively tight in the least. Especial pains should always be taken to double the blankets well around the feet. If the feet get warm readily, the patient generally comes out of the operation with agreeable feelings; but if they remain cold, the whole body feels uncomfortable a long time afterward. When the feet get warm with difficulty, a jug of hot water should be placed under them. The object of the wet sheet is never directly to excite sensible perspiration, as our author seems to suppose. The intention is to fill the superficial capillary vessels with blood, to develop the external or remote circulation, or, in other words, to produce a glow. The sensation of warmth should be the test for the time of remaining packed, not the perspirable or non-perspirable condition of the body.

THE SWEATING BLANKET—(AA.) Page 163.

Though this process was formerly resorted to very frequently, it is now seldom employed. Experience has proved that the other more mild and more agreeable processes, if the diet is plain and well regulated, will accomplish all that can be gained by forced sweating. Still there are a few cases, or rather conditions, in which it is decidedly advantageous. It is best adapted to persons of a gross, over-full habit of body, who require deterging pretty thoroughly. Gouty, rheumatic, and scrofulous subjects are most frequently in this condition. We should look to the state of the patient, rather than the name of the disease, in determining upon this process. During six years of water-cure practice, I have not used the dry sweating blanket in more than half a dozen cases. The dry packing is frequently serviceable to very feeble persons, who cannot exercise after a bath. In such cases it may follow the cold ablution, rubbing wet sheet, or wet pack, the patient remaining enveloped long enough to get up a comfortable glow. It is often useful, too, as a preparation for a cold bath of any kind, in those whose bodily temperature is low.

STIMULANTS AND TONICS—(BB.) Page 164.

These terms, in our hydropathic lexicon, have no particular meaning that I can discover. Their loose and indefinite employment in medical books is a source of endless confusion in ideas. In the allopathic technical sense, a stimulant is an article which produces a rapid and transient increase of vital energy (vital expenditure) and arterial action; a tonic produces the same effects more slowly, but they continue longer. Now these effects, called tonic and stimulant, are nothing more nor less than manifestations of the resistance of the organism to foreign and unnatural agents; hence, as all medical authors admit, the long-continued administration of any stimulant or tonic, though it is apparently strengthening at first, is invariably debilitating in the end. But the word stimulant, as generally employed in medical parlance, means an impression—any impression; in other words, any effect of any cause which excites vital action, or occasions vital disturbance, whether remedial or otherwise. Calomel, in medical writings, is sometimes called a stimulant, and sometimes a sedative; so of opium, and a hundred other things. Water-cure authors, in adopting the ambiguous language of the allopaths, have made some of their writings very absurd and contradictory. For example, Dr. E. Wilson says, in explaining the *modus operandi* of the hydropathic processes:

"There is one part of this process, however, that calls for special remark, and that is, the sudden immersion of the body in cold water while bathed with perspiration. This is easily explained; the skin is *stimulated* to excess, and were not some means taken to check the action, it would be prolonged indefinitely, and would be a cause of chill to the surface of the body, and give rise to cold and fever. The cold water applied in the manner described is a *stimulant;* it produces a momentary shock to the nervous system, causes the arrest of the perspiration, and is followed by a general reaction. In describing the manner in which cold was produced by draughts of cold air, I had occasion to remark that the checked perspiration was the effect, and not the cause, of the injury done to the system; and that the real cause of mischief was the chilling of the cutaneous nerves and the consequent depression of the nervous powers. *Cold never injures the body when acting as a stimulant;* it is only when it acts long upon the surface, and robs the latter of its heat."

Observe the incongruous senses in which the word stimulant is used, in the above quotation. In the first place, the skin is stimulated to excess by heat; this excessive stimulation is counteracted by the opposite stimulant of cold; and then we are told that a stimulant, as such, can never do any injury; but if the stimulation acts too long the body is injured, not by the stimulant, cold, but by being robbed of its heat, cold being the robber! Such reasoning is, simply, learned nonsense.

THE PLUNGE BATH—(CC.) Page 165.

By "more stimulating," the author means that the shock or impression is stronger. The plunge is one of the best baths on rising in the morning, as a hydroprophylactic measure. But, for the very reason that it is more shocking, I do not like it in fevers, especially those of nervous character. As a general rule, all those acute diseases, fevers, and inflammatory affections, in which the circulation is materially and continuously disturbed, and when, also, the nervous system is greatly exhausted, as in those forms of fever called typhoid, or nervous, are best treated by such applications as produce but a moderate first impression, as the wet rub sheet, packing sheet, ablutions, etc.

THE DOUCHE BATH—(DD.) Page 168.

Like the sweating blanket, the douche has been rather overdone at some of the establishments. Very nervous and irritable persons, and those subject to strong determinations to the brain, should always employ it cautiously, and with great moderation. For the majority of patients, from one to three minutes are amply sufficient. The best time for so powerful an application is when the stomach is nearly or quite empty; in the morning on rising, two to three hours after breakfast, and three to four hours after dinner.

WET BANDAGES—(EE.) Page 169.

The object of these can never be to "increase the heat of the stomach." The temperature of that organ is of no practical consequence. In all dyspeptic or debilitated stomachs, the vessels are relaxed, engorged, and overloaded. They have not sufficient contractile power to circulate their contents freely; hence accumulation, distension, congestion. A cold wet bandage, applied around the abdomen, operates on the double principle of direct and counter-irritation. The first impression excites the muscular fibres to contractile efforts, while that law of the animal economy which determines an increase of the circulating fluids to any point where an unnatural, unusual, or disproportionate impression is made, in some degree unloads the internal vessels, by calling more blood to the superficial. Whatever may be true or false in theory, none can dispute the great benefit derived from these appliances in all local diseases.

Constipation—(FF.) Page 171.

This is rather sophistical. The distinction attempted to be drawn between the agent producing an evil effect, and the said effect produced, is to my mind inconceivable. If a man is bled to death by the operation of venesection—a circumstance, by the way, not uncommon—it may as logically be said that the evil, death, was not so much from the agent, the lancet, as from the effect produced, viz., the bleeding.

In treating constipation hydropathically, more depends on the dietetic than on the bathing part of the management. I have never yet had a case to manage in which the bowels could not be brought to act regularly in a few days, and naturally in a few weeks. Months and years are sometimes required to remove all the distressing consequences of constipation and establish the general health; but I must think the motions of the bowels can, in all curable cases, be soon regulated by appropriate regimen. For food, unfermented wheat meal bread or biscuit, cracked wheat mush, boiled wheat, one or all should be prominent among the articles employed. Good, ripe, uncooked apples are excellent as part of the meal. Kneading, rubbing, thumping, and pounding, gently of course, the abdomen is a good exercise to promote free peristaltic action.

It is melancholy to reflect on the multifarious forms of disease which can be traced mainly to constipated bowels. Dyspepsia, liver complaints, nervous debility, hysteria, hypochondriasis, asthmatic and dropsical affections, cholera, colic, piles, skin diseases, etc., with their countless combinations and ramifications, may be generally traced to this starting point. Among our females who live in the ordinary way, scarcely one in a hundred is exempt from suffering on this account. The common primary cause is *concentrated food* and *mixed dishes.* Baker's bread, superfine flour in the shape of hot rolls, butter-biscuits, tea-cakes, short-cakes, etc., cause an immense amount of obstruction, debility, disease, and deformity. Under the general delusion that bran is a "mechanical irritant" or only food for horses and hogs, medical and non-medical people have rejected the very best part of their natural and healthful aliment. Mistaking sensuality for refinement, and man's depravity for God's intention, they have misimproved instead of bettering the order of nature, and dearly have they paid for the rash attempt.

When the cholera broke out in New York, in May last, our very learned and most egregiously mistaken Medical Council, Board of Health, and Sanatory Committee, by their official recommendations as to what the people should eat, drink, wear, and take as medicines, to prevent or ward off an attack, destroyed many more lives than they saved, if there is any truth in testimony. The whole sum and substance of their authoritative teaching was to induce people to use the most constipating kinds of food, and to resort to "checking" medicines on the appearance of any premonitory or suspicious symptom. Now it is a matter of plain common sense, as all will see, whose brains are not bewildered with the learned jargon of the doctors, that binding up the bowels with an unusual proportion of concentrated food and stimulants is exactly the way to produce obstruction, followed by inflammation, diarrhœa, and death. I have yet to learn of a single death among the thousands who pursued the contrary way—eating unconcentrated and *loosening* farinaceous food, with plenty of good fruits and vegetables.

FEVERS—(GG.) Page 172.

The hydropathic treatment of fevers is extremely simple, and has been, as far as I have been able to learn, uniformly successful. I have never heard of a fatal result when the patient was water-treated from first to last. Those who believe in the supremacy of drugs and destructives—supreme in mischief, I grant—may impute this success to the kind assistance of that singular deity who has been called chance. No matter. Chance never has and never will succeed as well on the other side. The number who have been treated for fevers of all kinds at water-cure establishments, and by water-cure practitioners in private practice, must amount to thousands. Is it not worth investigating why none of these have died? In my own practice I have treated continued, inflammatory, bilious, scarlet, typhus, and ship fevers, and in no case has the fever held out against the water appliances beyond the first week. The convalescence of a hydropathic patient contrasts advantageously with that of the half drugged-to-death subject of allopathic empyricism. He is never shattered, marred, or scarred in body, broken in constitution, nervous, preternaturally sensitive, full of aches and pains, ever liable to relapses, and constantly taking cold, as we know is the fact with many who recover from a fever *in spite* of the disease and the doctor both.

Non-professional persons who undertake the home-treatment of fevers are apt to do too much. The indications are—to allay the thirst by free water-drinking; to cleanse the bowels (when necessary) by copious water-injections, and to regulate the temperature by hot, warm, cool, or cold applications, generally or locally, according to the degree of heat. Cold ablutions, the wet sheet pack, or rubbing wet sheet, continued until the temperature becomes nearly natural, and repeated as often as it rises above the natural standard, will, in a few days at most, effect a subsidence of the general fever. If the feet incline to be cold, apply warm cloths or bottles of hot water; if any part is unnaturally hot, apply cold wet cloths frequently changed. Very long baths, or any strong applications which shock the system, I do not think desirable; nor do I believe exercise is to be recommended as a curative measure in any continued fever. Careful, gentle, quiet management, attending mainly to the regulation of the bodily temperature, is the best plan to treat all fevers.

As to food, the less the better, as a general rule, for the first few days. Until the violence of a fever is materially abated, the patient cannot digest, and burdening his stomach with food only adds to his troubles. It is a pernicious custom of the doctors and lay-folks—constantly stuffing the stomach of a fever patient with soups and slops, and toasts and teas. Let the stomach alone until it is capable of performing its digestive function. The appetite will then let you know it.

Gout and Rheumatism—(HH.) Page 173.

In treating these complaints, as far as sudorific processes are concerned, I would follow the rule previously intimated, which is applicable to all diseases alike—the condition of the body. I think the majority of gouty and rheumatic subjects will get thoroughly cured the soonest with but little sweating. I am in favor of what are sometimes called "long packs," in these complaints, where there are no strong determinations to the head or chest. The wet-sheet pack for an hour or an hour and a half, twice a day, followed by the plunge or douche, or a powerful shower, appears to me the best leading measure. All that the author recommends in respect to the management in other particulars, my experience fully endorses. There are no diseases in which out-door exercise, particularly walking, to the full extent of the patient's muscular ability, is more indispensable.

Inflammation of the Brain—(II.) Page 175.

I can see no necessity for shaving the head, or any part of it. Cold wet cloths can be changed once a minute, or oftener, if necessary; nor should we by any means wait twenty-four hours to see if favorable symptoms would not supersede the necessity of general treatment. We should *never* neglect general treatment a moment in any severe local inflammation. The wet sheets and general baths should be employed here precisely as in the case of simple fever; and all the rules applicable to the management of fevers will equally apply to all local inflammations. The only practical distinction is that something *additional* must be done to the seat of the local affection.

Inflammation of the Lungs—(JJ.) Page 176.

While discussing the pretensions of the hydropathic system with my whilom associates of the allopathic school, the question has more than once been asked me in seeming triumph, as though its very statement was a knock-down argument, "How would you treat pleurisy, or inflammation of the lungs?" The question is as easily answered as asked. And although I assure the orthodox gentlemen that I have been in the habit, for years, of treating all kinds of acute inflammatory affections of the chest, in men, women, and children, from sixty years of age down to six days, with hydropathy, and nothing else; although I aver that no one has ever died under such treatment, and notwithstanding I offer to give them name, place, time, and opportunity, they shake their full-stuffed heads dubiously, as much as to say, "There *must* be some mistake about it."

Here, as in all visceral inflammations, the general treatment is most important. Attend to the symptoms of fever as if it were *only* a fever; and apply wet bandages to the chest. Sitting and half baths, tepid or cold, according to the degree of *general* heat, are valuable auxiliaries to the wet-sheet packing.

Liver Complaints—(KK.) Page 178.

Acute inflammation of the liver is, in this climate, a very rare disease; hence the symptoms described in the text are not often recognized. What is known, or rather talked about and tampered with so much as "liver complaint," comprises various morbid conditions of that organ, as torpor, congestion, enlargement, induration, and chronic inflammation. For practical purposes, all those modifications of a morbid state may be regarded and treated as essentially the same. Imperfect functional action of the liver may emphatically be said to be the general condition consequent on the artificial habits of society. There are but few sound livers among us; in fact, the same affection has become general among our domesticated animals, resulting from the unnatural habits we have forced upon them.

There is an anatomical reason why the liver should be more liable to congestion and obstruction than any other organ in the body—liable, I mean, in reference to our improper habits. Unlike any other organ in the body, it is supplied with the venous or impure blood for its functional purposes. The venous or black blood from all parts of the body, charged with impurities, waste matters, and effete particles, passes on its way to the lungs for purification. A considerable portion of this blood is sent through the liver. This fact proves that the liver has much to do in relieving the blood of some of its useless and poisonous elements. If, then, the articles of our food and drink are impure, improper, or unnatural in any sense, the blood must become more loaded with effete matter than the various excretory organs can separate without their action being preternaturally increased. From the situation of the liver in relation to the venous circulation, it is at once manifest that it will be more readily overloaded with the floating impurities of the mass of blood than any other organ; and all experience corresponds with this fact. It is well known that fattened animals, hogs, cattle, poultry, kept on food to them unnatural and impure, almost invariably have diseased livers; and although these livers are very dainty dishes for human epicures to eat, these epicures must pardon me if I remind them that their own livers are in no bettêr condition, but rather worse.

In treating all the multitudinous ailments, commonly, and with about equal propriety, called "liver complaint," "dyspepsia," "nervous debility," "hypochondriasis," "jaundice," etc., a persevering course of the rubbing-wet sheet, wet-sheet pack, and sitz baths, are generally efficacious. Bad cases ought to remain under regular treatment one or two years. The diet should be strictly devoid of grease, condiments, and all concentrated aliments.

Cutaneous Eruptions—(LL.) Page 179.

The injury done to the constitution by repellent applications to the skin is not so well understood by the people as it ought to be. Washes made of different preparations of lead, and ointments of various preparations of mercury, constitute the regular orthodox prescriptions for almost all sorts of "breakings out" on the surface. These healing medicaments are pretty "sure cure," and exactly to the same extent *sure kill.* They do indeed smooth over the outside by repelling the disease to the internal mucous membrane. The following may serve to illustrate a principle of very general application: Once upon a time, I was consulted by a fond mother as to what she should do for her little boy's head. The child had an eruptive disease of the scalp, a mild form of *tinea capitis*, or scalled head. I answered, "Bathe it daily; give it no salt or grease to eat; keep the whole body healthy; let the eruption take care of itself; it does not look pretty, but it will disappear in due time; if you scatter it away with salves, ointments, or washes, it will show itself internally." My advice did not prevail; as usual in such cases a doctor was sent for who knew how to do something. He applied some sort of an "all-healing" ointment. The disease disappeared from the scalp and re-appeared on the mucous membrane of the windpipe, producing cough, and a hoarse, rough, croup-like sound of the voice, which may prove the germ of an early death from consumption.

Cholera and Bowel Complaints—(MM.) Page 181.

The cholera was treated in various parts of the United States hydropathically during its recent prevalence as an epidemic, and, as far as we have any account, with a success far beyond any other method employed. The management was considerably diversified by different practitioners. As a deduction from both theory and experience I am inclined to prefer, as a general rule, warm and tepid water internally to cold. In many cases, where there is great general heat, almost any quantity of cold water would be harmless. But in the majority of cases I think moderately warm water safer and more efficacious. On free drinking, and copious injections of warm or tepid water, I would place my main dependence, as far as local measures are concerned. For external applications I prefer cool or cold. The rubbing wet sheet, and wet-sheet pack have sometimes wonderfully re-established the external heat and circulation.

To bowel complaints generally, cholera morbus, cholera infantum, dysentery, and diarrhœa, all these remarks apply with equal force. The bowels should be promptly cleansed of all offending material by copious injections, repeated as often as the purging, griping, or other distressing symptoms demand. If there is much nausea, retchings, or vomiting, drink warm water freely until relief is obtained. Sitz baths and wet bandages are among the appliances which should not be neglected.

Nose Bleeding—(NN.) Page 181.

A method of arresting nasal hemorrhage, by compressing the upper lip, has lately been noticed in the medical journals. It is the discovery of an old shipmaster, whose process was to roll up a piece of paper and place it under the upper lip. Tying a knot in a bandage, and applying it on the upper lip, then fastening the bandage around the head has succeeded. The explanation is, that pressure on the upper lip compresses the artery furnishing the blood.

Condiments—(OO.) Page 191.

I cannot admire such reasoning. The same argument can be adduced with equal propriety in favor of tea, coffee, and tobacco. The idea that people who are enervated by a burning sun require stimulants, is a most palpable absurdity. They require exactly the contrary: the most rigid abstinence from every stimulating thing. It is the most common thing in the world for us erring mortals to mistake our own abuses for "gracious providences." "What did God make wine for, if not for us to enjoy?" asks the red-nosed critic, deeply steeped in alcoholic as well as theologic lore, in profound ignorance of the fact that God never made it at all! "What did God make hogs for, if not to eat?" exclaims the swine-loving sensualist. Pitiful humanity, that cannot perceive, in all the multitudinous tribes of animated nature, any higher motive of the Creator, than to pamper, brutalize, and sensualize his noblest workmanship—MAN!

LIQUORS, WITH THEIR EFFECTS, IN THEIR USUAL ORDER.

(SLIGHTLY ALTERED FROM J. C. LETTSOM, M.D.)

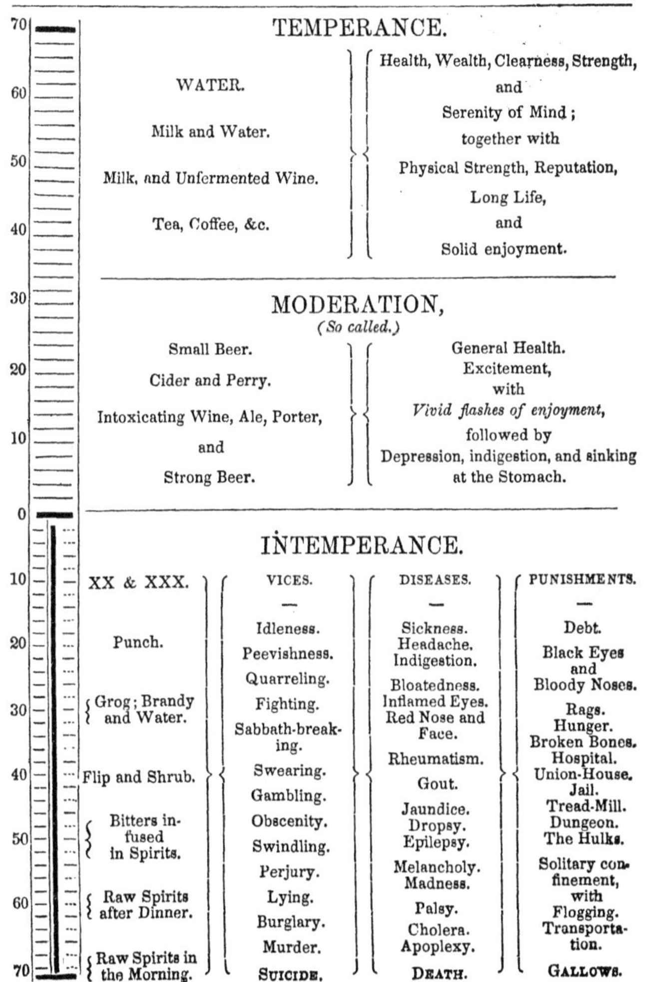

70

TEMPERANCE.

Liquors	Effects
WATER. Milk and Water. Milk, and Unfermented Wine. Tea, Coffee, &c.	Health, Wealth, Clearness, Strength, and Serenity of Mind; together with Physical Strength, Reputation, Long Life, and Solid enjoyment.

60 50 40 30

MODERATION,

(So called.)

Liquors	Effects
Small Beer. Cider and Perry. Intoxicating Wine, Ale, Porter, and Strong Beer.	General Health. Excitement, with *Vivid flashes of enjoyment,* followed by Depression, indigestion, and sinking at the Stomach.

20 10 0

INTEMPERANCE.

Scale	Liquors	VICES.	DISEASES.	PUNISHMENTS.
10	XX & XXX.	—	—	—
20	Punch.	Idleness. Peevishness. Quarreling.	Sickness. Headache. Indigestion. Bloatedness.	Debt. Black Eyes and Bloody Noses.
30	Grog; Brandy and Water.	Fighting. Sabbath-breaking.	Inflamed Eyes. Red Nose and Face. Rheumatism.	Rags. Hunger. Broken Bones. Hospital.
40	Flip and Shrub.	Swearing. Gambling.	Gout.	Union-House. Jail.
50	Bitters infused in Spirits.	Obscenity. Swindling. Perjury.	Jaundice. Dropsy. Epilepsy. Melancholy. Madness.	Tread-Mill. Dungeon. The Hulks. Solitary confinement,
60	Raw Spirits after Dinner.	Lying. Burglary. Murder.	Palsy. Cholera. Apoplexy.	with Flogging. Transportation.
70	Raw Spirits in the Morning.	SUICIDE.	DEATH.	GALLOWS.

INDEX.

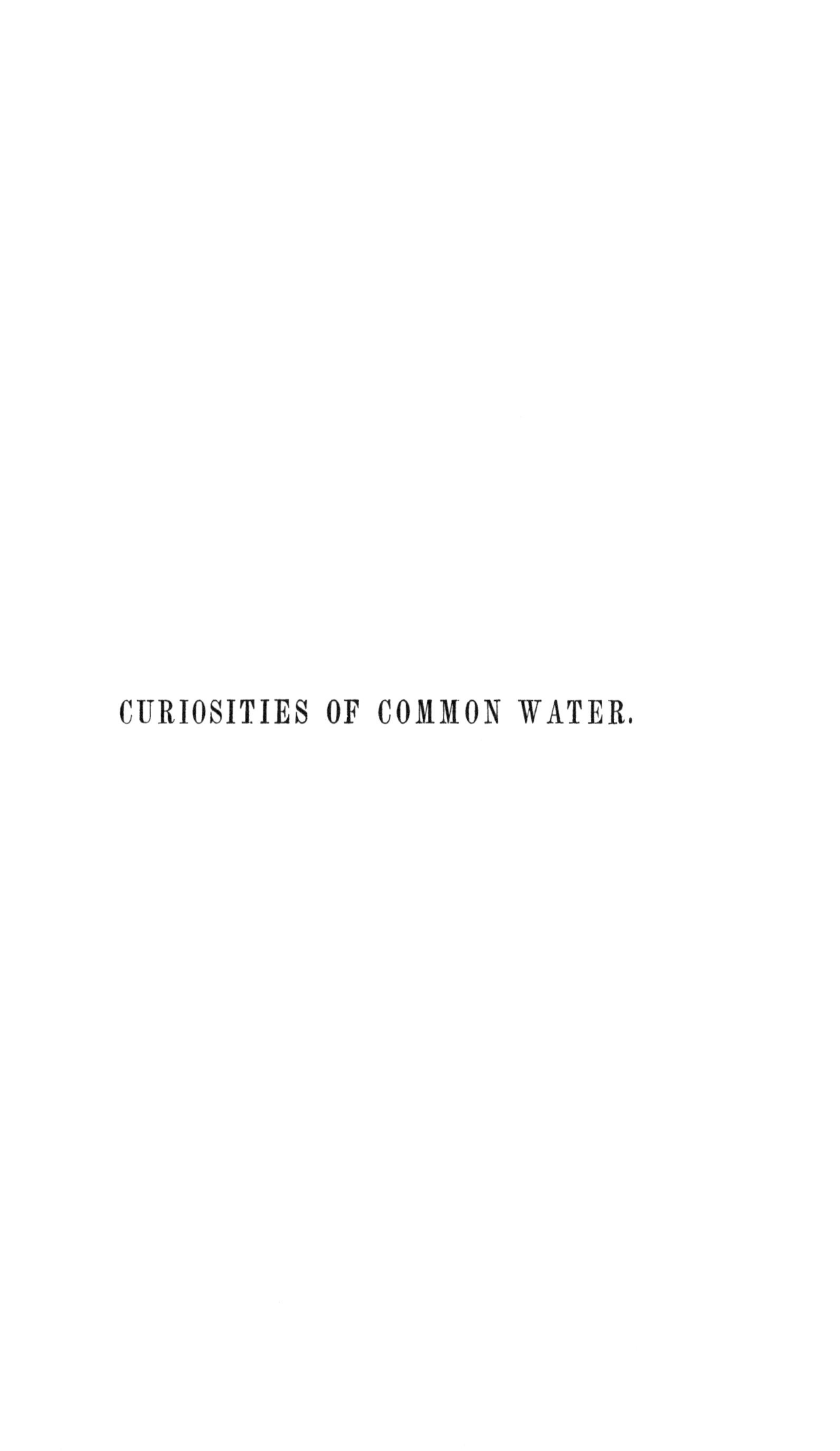

CURIOSITIES OF COMMON WATER.

CURIOSITIES

OF

COMMON WATER:

OR,

THE ADVANTAGES THEREOF IN

PREVENTING AND CURING MANY DISEASES.

GATHERED FROM

THE WRITINGS OF SEVERAL EMINENT PHYSICIANS, AND ALSO FROM MORE THAN FORTY YEARS' EXPERIENCE.

BY JOHN SMITH, C. M.

TO WHICH ARE ADDED

Some Rules for Preserving Health by Diet.

That's the best physic which doth cure our ills
Without the charge of 'pothecaries' bills.

FROM THE FIFTH LONDON EDITION, 1723.

WITH ADDITIONS BY JOEL SHEW, M. D.

STEREOTYPED.

NEW YORK:
FOWLERS AND WELLS, 131 NASSAU STREET.
LONDON:
C. DONOVAN, 7 KING WILLIAM STREET.
1849.

Entered, according to Act of Congress, in the year 1849,
BY FOWLERS AND WELLS,
in the Clerk's Office of the District Court for the Southern District of New York.

BANER & PALMER, STEREOTYPERS,
201 William street, corner of Frankfort, N. Y.

PREFACE.

It is sometimes said by objectors to the modern water-cure, that the system is no new thing; that water has always been regarded as one of the best of all remedial agents; and that therefore it is a fallacy to set up a claim for a new system, the great remedial agent of which is as old as any other known. But it need only be remarked in reference to this pretended objection, that every advocate of the modern water-treatment claims for water *antiquity in its use.* The objection, therefore, has no weight.

The following work, copied from the fifth London edition, of 1723, is a proof that the virtues of simple water were better known at that period than at a much later date. The work is a valuable one, and in the hands of our energetic publishers, will be the means of doing at least some good, which is more than can be said of a majority of books now-a-days published.

The additions we have made are included in brackets, and may thus be easily distinguished from the body of the original work.

With the full belief that this work will prove useful to many who are personally interested in the subject of health, it is given to the American public.

J. S.

New York, 1849.

THE

CURIOSITIES OF COMMON WATER.

For the benefit of mankind in general, I have taken pains to give the world an account of what I have found written in the works of the most eminent physicians, concerning the good that mankind may receive from the use of common water; and of the information I have had concerning the benefits thereof from others by word of mouth; and of what I have discovered by my own experience, from frequent trials during a time that hath intervened from that of thirty to seventy-four years of age; which is sufficient to confirm the stupendous effects thereof in many particulars, that shall be mentioned as my own discovery with respect to this excellent remedy, which will perform cures with very little trouble, and without any charge, and is also to be had wherever there are any habitations, which is what can hardly be said of any other thing. So that in some sense, water may be truly styled an universal remedy, since the diseases it either prevents or cures may have this remedy applied to all persons, and in all places where men do inhabit.

EXCELLENCY OF WATER.

The first commendation of common water that I shall mention, is that which is written concerning it by Dr. Manwaring, in his Method and Means of enjoying

Health, wherein he saith, that water is a wholesome drink, or rather the most wholesome, being appointed for man in his best state; which doth strongly argue that drink to be the most suitable for human nature, answering all the intentions of common drinks, for it cools, moistens, and quencheth thirst; it is clear, thin, and fit to convey the nourishment through the smallest vessels of the body, and is a drink that is a rule to itself, and requires little caution in the use of it, since none will be tempted to drink of it more than needs; and that in the primitive ages of the world, water-drinkers, he says, were the longest livers by some hundreds of years, nor so often sick and complaining as we are.

Dr. Keill, when he treats concerning the stomach, in his Abridgment of the Anatomy of Human Bodies, saith, that water seems the fittest to promote digestion of the food which we eat; all spirituous liquors having a property by which they hurt rather than help digestion, the sad effects of which they are sensible of, he saith, who, by a long use thereof, have lost their appetites, hardly ever to be restored without drinking water, which seldom faileth of procuring a good appetite and a strong digestion. With which Dr. Baynard does agree in that affirmation, "that water liquefies and concocts our food better than any fomented liquor whatever."—*Hist. of Cold Bathing*, p. 440.

Dr. Prat, in his Treatise of Mineral Waters, shows it to be his judgment, that if people would accustom themselves to drink water, they would be more free from many diseases, such as tremblings, palsies, apoplexies, giddiness, pains in the head, gout, stone, dropsy, rheumatism, piles, and such like; which diseases are most common among them that drink strong drinks, and which water generally would prevent. Moreover, he also saith, that water plentifully drank, strengthens the stomach, causeth an appetite, preserves the sight, maketh the senses lively, and cleanseth all the passages of the body, especially those of the kidneys and bladder.

It is also said by Dr. Duncan, in his Treatise of Hot Liquors, that when men contented themselves with water they had more health and strength; and that at this day those who drink nothing but water are more healthy, and live longer than those who drink strong liquors, which raises the heat of the stomach to excess, whereas water keeps it in a due temper. And he adds in another part of the book, that by hot liquor the blood is inflamed; and such whose blood is inflamed live not so long as those who are of a cooler temper. A hot blood being commonly the cause of fluxes, rheums, ill digestion, pains in the limbs, headache, dimness of sight, and especially of hysteric vapors. He also imputes the cause of ulcers to a hot blood, and declares, that if men kept their blood cool and sweet by a moderate and cooling diet, they would never be troubled with ulcers or other breakings-out. Which coolness of the blood will be well performed by drinking a large draught of water in the morning, which will carry off the bilious and salt recrements by urine. And if water is drank also after dinner, it will cool a hot stomach, and prevent the rising of those fermentations which cause winds and belching after meat, so that if persons who are liable to these disorders, will leave off strong liquors and a hot diet, and drink water, they will procure better health to themselves than they had before.

Sir John Floyer, also, in his Treatise of Cold Baths, does affirm (p. 109, edition 5), that water-drinkers are temperate in their actions, prudent, and ingenious; they live safe from those diseases which affect the head; such as apoplexies, palsies, pain, blindness, deafness, gout, convulsions, trembling, madness; and the drinking of water cures the hiccough, fœtor of the mouth, and of the whole body; it resists putrefaction, and cools burning heats and thirsts, and after dinner it helps digestion. And if the virtues of cold water were seriously considered, all persons would value it as a great medicine, in preventing the stone, asthma, and hysteric fits; and to the use of this children ought to be bred up from their cradles. And in page 434 he saith, that as water is in chief the universal drink of the world, so it is the best and most salubrious. And in page 437, that he hath known where a regular drinking of spring water hath done considerable cures, by washing off the acrid, scorbutic salts from the blood, and strengthening the coats and fibres of the stomach and bowels, and hath brought on a good appetite and strong digestion.

[Sir John Floyer also says: "That good pure water has a *balsamic* and healing quality in it, I could give many instances, as well externally in curing wounds, as internally in ulcers, excoriations, etc., for I once knew a gentleman of plentiful fortune, who by some accident fell to decay, and, having a numerous family of small children, while the father was a prisoner at the King's Bench, his family was reduced almost to want, his wife and children living on little other than bread and water. But I never saw such a change in six months, as I did in this unhappy family; for the children that were always ailing and valetudinary, as with coughs, king's evil, etc., were recovered to a miracle, looked fresh, well colored, and lusty, their flesh hard and plump."]

Having read over an old book, written by one Sir Thomas Elliot, entitled The Castle of Health, he there declared from his own experience, that in the county of Cornwall, though it was a very cold quarter, the poorer sort, which in his time did never, or but very seldom, drink any other drinks but water, were strong of body and lived to a very great age; to which relation that of Sir Henry Blount is very agreeable, who affirmed in his book of Travels into the Levant (where, under the Turkish government, the use of wine was forbid, and where the common drink is water), that he then had a better stomach to his food, and digested it more kindly than he ever did before or since.

And in the Treatise of the Vanity of Philosophy, written by Dr. Gideon Harvey, it is affirmed by him, that it is not heat that causeth a good digestion, but a proper ferment, or liquor, provided by nature, to dissolve the food into a substance like unto pap made with fine flour, which dissolvent, he saith, is much depraved by hot spirituous liquors; and therefore he commends water above all other drinks to promote digestion.

[Hahn, a German physician, says: "Water does not, as some suppose, weaken the stomach, but increases the appetite, as may be seen by the larger quantity of food taken at meals. Those who make this assertion contradict themselves; for a debilitant stomach requires a less, and not a larger quantity of food. Others imagine that by drinking water they lose their color and flesh. Even if this were the case, and they did become a little paler and thinner, such a loss is not to be compared with the general improvement of health which is obtained thereby. It yet remains to be shown, whether a protuberant stomach, with swollen, flabby, puffed-out cheeks, is to be preferred to a more slender shape, and a thinner face; or whether the rude country glow of health, with rosy cheeks, is not to be preferred to that pale and sickly hue so much admired by people of fashion. But water-drinkers generally retain their flesh and healthy color. A few, however, who had swollen, flabby, or spongy flesh, and therefore unhealthy, have in appearance become thinner, and lost their puffiness, having exchanged it for a firm and compact flesh, therefore healthy. Those who, from the use of ardent spirits and thick, glutinous beverages, as beer, brandy, etc., have got reddened, violet copper-colored faces, have not by drinking water become pale, but have exchanged their violet or purple redness for a more natural color. Every man, I think, ought to be satisfied with such a change."

Dr. Cheyne, of Dublin, says: "I had once the opportunity of inquiring into the habits of the workmen of a large glass factory. They generally wrought from twenty-four to thirty-six hours at a time, according as the furnace continued in a proper state, and I found during this time, which was technically called a journey, that to supply the waste caused by perspiration, they drank a large quantity of water, in the quality of which they were very curious; it was the purest and softest water in the district, and was brought from a distance of two miles. There were three men out of more than one hundred, that drank nothing but water; the rest drank porter or ardent spirits. The three water-drinkers appeared to be of their proper age, while the rest, with scarcely an exception, seemed ten or twelve years older than they proved to be."

The editor of the London Lancet, about four years since, said: "If we could always persuade a patient who consults us for the first fit of the gout, to arınk water for the rest of his life, to take exercise, and to diminish by half the amount of animal food he is in the habit of taking, there would be but little chance of a return of the attack."

Zimmerman, the author of the well-known work on Solitude, and physician to Frederick the Great, king of Prussia, strongly recommended water. "Water," says he, "does not chill the ardor of genius." He instances Demosthenes, whose sole drink was water. "Pure soft water is the most suitable drink for man."]

GOUT AND HYPOCHONDRIAC MELANCHOLY

Water-drinking is also said by Dr. Allen to be good to prevent two deplorable distempers; the gout and the hypochondriac melancholy. For, says he, the gout is generally caused by the too great drinking of fermented liquors, and is never said to have assaulted any drinker of water; and he saith also, that melancholy hypochondria is kept off longest by drinking water instead of strong drink. To which let me add, that I once knew a gouty gentleman, who, to avoid his drinking companions in London, retired to New Brentford, where I then lived; in which town, by a very temperate diet of one meal a day, and drinking only water, he lived two whole years free from pain. But being visited by one who came that way, and invited to drink but one bottle of claret between them, he fell next day into a terrible fit of the gout, which held above a month after; of which being recovered, he, by the same course, continued well till I left the place, which was about a year and a half after.

WATER PREVENTS THE GRAVEL.

The good properties of water are further manifested in preventing the breeding of gravel in the kidneys; for Zechias, in Consult. 17, as he is quoted by Salmon, affirms, that nothing does so much abate the heat of the kidneys, and free them from those recrements which cause pain in the back, one great sign of gravel, as water does; but he adviseth to drink it warm, by the use of which, he saith, the unnatural heat in time will be so extinguished, that no more of that matter causing gravel will be produced in the body. Which assertion by experience I have found to be true; for observing much gravel to be voided by me, as also abundance of matter floating in the urine like bran, with a great number of recrements like cuttings of hair, some above an inch long, which substances were found in all the water that I made in above twelve months, for which I could get no remedy, I was advised to drink water, which in about half a year did entirely free me from those symptoms, which some out of ignorance imputed to witchcraft, so that from that time to this present I never have been troubled with it.

STONE IN THE BLADDER.

Water also is commended as efficacious to prevent the breeding of the stone in the bladder, for it hath been observed that in some who have been cut for the stone, that new stones have been engendered, so that some young persons have been cut several times. Now to prevent this, the drinking of water hath been advised with success; for by this that intemperate heat in the body was abated, which did occasion the distemper. Some have advised to drink it warm, and others cold, and in particular, Van Heydon, a physician of Ghent, in Flanders, in his book, entitled "Help for the Rich and Poor;" which, he saith, in p. 49, is sufficiently insinuated by Piso and Alexander, who do assure us, that the taking a draught of cold water in the morning hath done so much good, that several, after the voiding of a stone, never had any more stones grow in them.

Which experiment may give light to the discovery of a way to cure the stone without cutting; for if the growing of new stones can be prevented by drinking water, let it be hot or cold, it may prevent a stone from growing bigger when begun; and if the adding matter to increase a stone new begun, can be prevented, nature in time may waste that which is begun, especially if some drops of sweet spirit of nitre be added to all the water drank, which will powerfully help to cool, and is known to be an admirable mover or provoker of urine, and will waste a stone, and make it crumble like fuller's earth, if applied to a stone taken from the body. Or the water may be sweetened with honey, which is now much in use among the gentry, as I am informed by an ingenious apothecary; who told me that among them at present, pump-water and honey was in great repute to give ease in gravel: and there is so near an affinity between gravel and the stone, that what is proper for one will be suitable to both, and will prevent the growing of both.

WATER BENEFICIAL IN CHILD-BEARING.

Water is also styled in Sennertus's works, the balsam of children, the drinking of it by the mother being one of those things whereby children may be strengthened in the womb, and will prevent those injuries that are done them by drinking strong liquors; which Sampson's mother was not allowed to do, for she was commanded not to drink wine or strong drink.—Judg. xiii. 4. But I will not say, if all women should do this, their children shall be as strong as Sampson was; yet this I will say, if they would do this, they would find their children more free from diseases and frowardness, and so much more easy to nurse and bring up, and be less liable to an immature death; the want of which abstinence from strong drinks is the cause why so many rich people find it hard to bring up children, in comparison to what is done by the poor; for these last are born of mothers who not only are prevented from being gluttons by their want of dainties, which are deceitful meat (Prov. xxiii. 3), but they seldom taste wine or strong drink; whereas, the rich not only feed high, but they also drink strong drinks, which in most constitutions do overheat and corrupt the humors of the body, and that blood by which their children are nourished during pregnancy. Which injury to unborn infants would be prevented, if the mother would be temperate in diet, and drink water, especially at meals, by which the blood of the mother would be kept cool and clean; which must needs communicate a healthful substance to the child within her, and prevent all those distempers which infants do bring with them into the world.

WATER INCREASES MILK IN WOMEN.

And here it may be proper to add, what by divers experiments hath been found to be true, that the drinking water by nurses while they give suck to children, will wonderfully increase milk in those that want it, as every one will find, who can be persuaded to make use thereof. I have advised many to make use of it, who have found that by drinking a large draught of water at bed-time, they have been supplied with milk sufficient for that night, when before, they wanted it and could not be supplied by any other means: and besides, they who have found their children restless, by reason of too much heat in their milk, do find them much more quiet after their milk is cooled by water-drinking.

WATER STAYS HUNGER.

By drinking water also, the want of food for a time may be suffered without starving; for I have been informed by a credible friend, who was an officer at sea, that being sent down to Stafford to take care to see some men conveyed on shipboard, that had been pressed by act of Parliament for the sea-service, he found in the prison where they were kept, a lusty fellow, who had declared he would starve himself rather than go to sea; and taking particular notice thereof, he found upon due inquiry, that for twenty days he had refused to eat any manner of food, only he drank each day about three pints or two quarts of water, hoping thereby to get himself discharged: but when he found his pretensions to be in vain, and that in about two days they should all march for London, he condescended to eat some food, beginning with a little, and in the march he was observed to travel as well as the best man. I find also an account in Dr. Car's letters, of a certain crack-brained man, who, at Leyden, when the doctor resided in that university, pretended he could fast as long as Christ did; and it was found that he held out the time of forty days without eating any food, only he drank water and smoked tobacco. And I once had a sad complaint from a poor old woman of the greatness of her want, affirming that oftentimes she had not eaten any food for two or three days; upon which I asked her, if she did not then suffer much uneasiness in her stomach? She said she did; but found a way at last to assuage her hunger by drinking water, which did satisfy her appetite.

[The living body may be compared to a perpetual furnace, which has a tendency constantly, by evaporation, to become dry. Its natural temperature internally, 98° Fahrenheit, is much above that of the surrounding objects of nature, and hence this result. If all food and water are for a length of time withheld from the animal, he becomes parched and feverish; in a few days, at most, delirium supervenes, and if the experiment be continued any considerable time, death is the inevitable result. A human being dies in about three weeks without food or water; but if the indication of thirst is answered by a free supply of pure soft water, the individual lives more than twice that length of time.

In the "Transactions of the Albany Institute," for 1830, Dr. McNaughton relates the case of one Reuben Kelsey, a religious maniac, twenty-seven years of age, who lived on water alone for fifty-three days. The first six weeks he was able to walk out every day, and sometimes spent a great part of the day in the woods.

His walk was said to be steady and firm, and his friends even remarked that his step had an unusual elasticity. He shaved himself until about a week before his death, and was able to sit up in bed to the last day. And in the Boston Medical and Surgical Journal, Dec. 13, 1848, Dr. W. V. Edmonson, of East New Market, Md., gives an account of a gentleman of that vicinity, aged eighty-five years, who had lived, eschewing all nourishment except air and water, for forty-three days and five hours. His bowels were moved the first twenty days, once; the next fifteen days, twice; the remaining eight days, three times. He had been indisposed some ten days prior to the period of fasting. He was a man of industrious habits, frugal, and temperate.]

WATER STRENGTHENS WEAK CHILDREN.

Water is also of great use to strengthen weak children, for we are informed by Dr. Joseph Browne, in his treatise of cures performed by cold baths, that the Welsh women do preserve their children from the rickets, by washing them night and morning in cold water, till they are three quarters of a year old (p. 79). And it is said by Sir John Floyer, in his treatise of cold baths, that a lady in Scotland, who had lost several children through weakness, did, by the advice of a highland beggar woman, preserve those she had afterward, by washing them daily in cold water. And I myself did advise a neighbor, whose child began to be rickety, to treat the child in the same manner; but she, instead of washing, dipped it over head and ears every morning, it being then in the summer time: the event of which was, the child became strong, and had a good countenance, though before, it was in the face very pale and wan. Which shows how great the power of water is, when used outwardly to invigorate the spirits, and strengthen nature.

[Sir John Floyer says: "It is a Welsh saying, '*that no child has the rickets unless it has a dirty slut for a nurse.*'"

Sudden cold immersions, in cases of infants and chil dren suffering from rickets, was long a favorite remedy with the English. Dr. Baynard wrote, in 1706, as follows, concerning the *causes* of rickets: "As to the rickets, it was a distemper in England almost worn out, but now it begins to come in play again. But in the time of King Charles I., it was almost epidemical, few families escaping it; especially those that were rich and opulent, and put their children out to nurse; where, through unnatural usage, and vicious, disagreeable milk, the infant was soon spoiled by contracting from the drunken nurse, cacocymious juices; hence, with the growing infant, grew up the boot fashion for the men, and long coats for the women; for they were so ashamed at their crooked legs, that they wore boots to hide them. And this beginning at court (among the gentry), the straight-legged fools must follow the fashion, and wear boots too, with great boot-hose tops of fine linen, laced, etc., and jingling spurs, which gave occasion to the then witty Spanish ambassador at his return home, to jest upon our follies; for being asked by his master, the Spanish king, if London were a populous city? he answered it was. 'Was!' replied the king; 'why, is it not so now?' 'No,' quoth the ambassador, 'I believe they are gone ere this, for they were all booted before I came out of town.'

"These nurses spoil and destroy, through neglect and

want of (true mother) tenderness, two thirds of the poor infants committed to their care. A very pious and good man, minister at this time of a certain town not far from London, on the banks of the river of Thames, told me, with a great deal of sorrow and concern, that it was the greatest trouble he had in the world to see, even in his own parish, how many children were sacrificed yearly to the barbarous treatment and ill usage of their nurses, what with bad milk of their own, and feeding the young infant with mixed meats and drinks, as yeasty new ale, or stale beer, etc., which makes it puke, or gives it the gripes, from green, porraceous bile, etc. Then it has the worms, forsooth, and must be physicked the nurse's way, by some neighboring drunken old woman, or favorite quack or apothecary, who vouches for the nurse's care, that its time was come, and no more could be done; and this dismal alarm is posted to the parents two hours after it is dead, to haste down, the child being suddenly taken very ill, and that usually when it is overlaid, or choaked with hard bandage, etc. Down comes madam, the mother, furbelowed, with an erected rump (crying and bellowing), and running about half mad, like a cow stung with a gad-fly, and with her maid laden with pots, glasses, Venice-treacle, goody Kent's powder, goat-stone, black-cherry-water, etc. And after her, Easie, her husband, with a coach-and-four, and perhaps a brace of doctors, or some famous child's apothecary, etc. And thus the parents are kept in the dark, and the murder of their children stifled, when all this might have been avoided, by bringing the child up by hand, at home, under the mother's eye, if through weakness, or want of milk or good nipples, she could not nurse it herself."]

SWELLINGS FROM BRUISES.

It is also a known custom, to prevent the swellings that follow bruises in the faces of children, by immediately applying thereunto a linen cloth, four or six times double, dipped in cold water, and new dipping it as it begins to grow warm; for the cold repels or prevents the flowing of humors to the part, which otherwise would cause great swelling, and after turn blackish. And if, upon neglecting to do so, a swelling should succeed, it may be discussed by fomenting night and morning, for an hour at a time, with water as hot as can be endured; for that will give vent to the humors to transpire through the skin, or dissolve them, so as to make them capable of returning back.

SICKNESS AT THE STOMACH AND VOMITING BY WATER.

Moreover, by means of water all sickness at the stomach may be cured, which is done thus: Take four quarts of water, make it as hot over the fire as you can drink it; of which water let a quart be taken down at several draughts; then wrap a rag round a small piece of stick, till it is about the bigness of a man's thumb; tie it fast with some thread; and with this, by endeavoring gently to put it a little way down your throat, provoke yourself to vomit up again most of the water; then drink another quart and vomit up that, and repeat the same the third and fourth time. You may also provoke vomiting by tickling your throat with your finger, or the feather-end of a goose-quill; but the cloth round a skewer maketh one vomit with most ease, which is done with no trouble when the stomach is full. And by this way of vomiting, which will be all performed in an hour's time, that vicious and ropy phlegm in the stomach, which causeth the sickness, will be cast up, so that the party in that time will be free from all that inward disturbance, if you use the remedy at first; but if the sickness hath continued for a time, it will require the same course once or twice more, which may be done in three or four hours, one after another, without any other inconvenience, besides that of being a little sore in the breast the next day, which will soon go off by the force of nature. Which remedy, by forty years' experience, I look upon to be infallible in all sickness at the stomach, from what cause soever, and for all pains in the belly which seem to be above the navel; for these are all in the stomach, as by long experience I have found: which pains are generally counted the colic; but it is not so; for true colics are always below the navel, in the large intestine, or colon. And by this means I have eased very great pains, caused by eating muscles that were poisonous; and it is also a certain cure for all surfeits or disorders that follow after much eating; so that the lives of multitudes might be saved by this means, who, for want of expelling what offends, do often die in misery. For, by thus cleansing the stomach at the first, the root of diseases proceeding from surfeiting, or unwholesome food, or any vicious humors from a bad digestion, are prevented; the stomach being the place in which all distempers do at first begin. No man was more subject to sickness than myself before thirty years of age; but since I found out the way of vomiting with water, which is now above forty years, I never have been sick for two days together; for when I find myself ill to any great degree, I betake myself to this way of vomiting, which in an hour's time restores me to ease, and perfectly removes my illness. And the same benefit all my family find in it, as do others also, whom I can persuade to try the experiment; which is such, that no physician whatever can advise a better to the king himself, should he fall sick. For, in the first place, it is not a nauseous remedy—it does not make the patient sick, as the best of all other vomits do; and then it is a vomit which is at our own command, since we can leave off when we please; and it infallibly works a cure to all sick stomachs.

Some few, indeed, pretend they are not able to vomit by this means. Now, if they cannot vomit, let them take a pint of water, when they find themselves ill from eating, and do so every three or four hours, eating no more till they are hungry; and they will find the water digest and carry off what was offensive. The ingenious Dr. Cheyne, in his Treatise of the Gout, doth affirm, that warm water drank freely in a morning fasting, and at meals (and I say cold water is as good), hath been a sovereign remedy for restoring lost appetites, and strengthening weak digestions, when other more pompous medicines have failed. And he adviseth gouty persons, after excess either in meat or drink, to swill down as much fair water as their stomachs will bear, before they go to bed, whereby they will reap these advantages—either the contents of the stomach will be thrown up, or both meat and drink will be much diluted, and the labor and expense of spirits in digestion much saved. And indeed I have found, by long experience, that nothing causeth so good a digestion as fair water; but this requires time to free us from the uneasiness that an ill digestion causeth, whereas vomiting is an immediate remedy, and frees a man from it upon the spot.*

* At sea, on our homeward passage from England, ship Switzerland, Captain E. Knight, November 29th, 1846, I was informed that Mrs. W——, a worthy English woman, with a young infant at the breast, wished me to see her in the steerage. I found her writhing and groaning with cramp in the stomach; the extremeties were cold and the surface pale. She could not lie, but was in a sitting posture, held by assistants. The wind was howling through the shrouds, and the motion of the vessel so great that one was compelled to lay hold of any thing near in order to stand. I inquired whether Mrs. W—— had been eating any thing that disagreed, when I was told that her bowels had been out of order for some days. She had lately taken her meals irregularly, and this day, particularly, her food had gone badly. She ate about evening, and this had made her worse; then, in about an hour, a kind-hearted old gentleman prepared a nice dish of coffee, with spices in it, which he thought would do her good. This, of course, only made her the worse.

The treatment in such cases is simple and easily understood. According to the old mode of practice, some would adopt the plan of giving an emetic, tartarized antimony, ipecac, the sulphates of copper or zinc, flour of mustard, or perhaps, what would be least harmful and most efficient of all these, lobelia inflata. By such means the patient may often be relieved; but it is always at the expense of injury to the stomach—an evil, greater or less, which should, if possible, be avoided. If the patient is a short, thick-necked, fat person, and something advanced in years, bleeding would be practiced before giving the emetic, with the view of preventing apoplexy. Others, again, would give large doses of some opiate, solid opium, or, what would act more quickly, laudanum in very large doses, as forty, fifty, or even sixty drops, often repeated till the effect is produced. Those who have undergone any of these (to us terrible modes), and have also tested the effects of water-treatment in like cases, can judge as to which are best.

I told Mrs. W—— I should treat her differently from what she had been accustomed to, but would do precisely as if myself were in her case. I at once ordered an abundance of water, about blood-warm, to make it as mawkish as might be. She then drank, at my direction, as quickly as possible, a number of tumblers, and instantly copious vomiting took place. A large amount of acid and undigested matters was thrown off. She drank and vomited again and again, till the stomach became thoroughly cleansed. The pain subsided, and she went to rest; the feet were rubbed, and a bottle of moderately warm water was placed to them, and she soon slept. Next day she nearly fasted, taking only a little water-gruel. She had no pain, grew stronger, and in every respect better.

We are told by Sir John Floyer, in his Treatise of Bath and Mineral Springs, that vomiting with water is very useful in the gout, sciatica, flatulency, shortness of breath, hypochondriac melancholy, and falling sickness; which distempers are usually derived from evil matter contained in the stomach, as is likewise giddiness in the head, and apoplexies, with which myself once seemed to be threatened; for, after eating a plentiful dinner, I was seized with giddiness, and the sight of my eyes became so depraved, that things seemed double, which was accompanied by a strange consternation of spirit; and having read that apoplexies generally seize after eating, I immediately called for water, and not daring to stay till it was warmed, I drank it cold, and by the help of my finger provoked vomiting, upon which I did immediately overcome the evils I was threatened with; the symptoms before mentioned being the same as did precede the fit of an apoplexy in another person, as himself afterward told me, who died of it the third fit, about a year after.

WATER IN SHORTNESS OF BREATH.

As for people who are troubled with shortness of

She omitted tea and coffee, and was careful in diet, exercised on deck in the open air, and thus grew better and better the whole passage.

In some cases of this kind it is necessary, besides the vomiting, to give injections. There is no danger of vomiting and purging too much, provided the water is pure, and used neither too cold nor hot. Quart after quart of lukewarm injections may be given, until the alimentary canal is thoroughly cleansed, and the pain removed. Frictions upon the bowels, woolen cloths, or towels, wrung out of warm water, and the like, may be resorted to. I have never, in one instance, failed soon to bring relief in these cases. Once in a hundred, spasm may be so severe that the wet sheet will be needed before complete relief can be obtained. Mark well the very small amount only of food allowable for some days after attacks of this kind.—*Water-Cure Manual, by Joel Shew, M. D.*

breath, it is certain from experience, that vomiting with warm water three or four times will afford certain relief. And the same may be prevented by drinking nothing but water afterward, either cold, or warmed with a toast; for upon doing this, the difficulty of breathing will apparently abate; which water, if you please, may be boiled with honey. And I knew one who, by this means, as he was advised by me, lived comfortably in this city two or three winters; but, having undertaken business which did occasion drinking strong drinks, was the next winter carried off by the distemper; wine, ale, and brandy, being as bad as poison to people troubled with shortness of breath. So that nothing but water ought to be drank in that distemper.

WATER PREVENTS VOMITING AND CHOLERA MORBUS.

Some people are taken with violent vomiting, and the excess thereof in some hath been so great as to endanger their lives—yea, cause death: in which case water will be very helpful; for if a pint of it warmed be drank after every vomit, it will prevent that violent straining, wherein lieth the danger of all vomiting, because to strain violently, when but little will come up, does endanger the breaking of some inward vessel. And besides this, the offending matter will be sooner loosened from the internal part of that bowel, the stomach, and cast out, upon which the vomiting will sooner cease. For after this manner the famous Sydenham, a most honest writer, did overcome the cholera morbus, or vomiting and looseness, so common in his time, and was found by the weekly bill to kill more than now die of convulsions; for his way was to boil a chicken in four gallons of water, which made a broth not much differing from water, of which he ordered large draughts to be given, and some of it to be taken by clyster, till the whole quantity was spent, if the vomiting did not stop before; which did so take off the sharpness of the matter offending, and wash it out, that the party in a little time became well. And the same was the practice of Sigismundus Grasius, who commends pure water, in a vomiting and looseness, to be drank in large quantities; for thereby, he saith, the corrosive and sharp humors will be so weakened, that they will no more offend. And, he saith, it may be drank cold, if the patient be strong; otherwise let it be warmed.

FLUXES.

And in common fluxes without vomiting, a quart or more of warm water drank, will so weaken the sharpness whereby the distemper is caused, that it will soon be overcome, and the gripings eased; and in the bloody flux, which is the most dangerous of all fluxes, the ingenious Cornelius Celsus adviseth a large drinking of cold water as the best of remedies: but then no other substance must be taken till the disease is cured. And another great physician, by name Lusitanus, affirms (Cent. I. Obser. 46), "that he knew one, who, being in the summer time afflicted with the bloody flux, did drink a large quantity of cold water, and did thereby recover. This large quantity of water, therefore, in these fluxes, doth so correct the sharpness of the humor offending, that it can have no power to cause pain, or corrode the vessels, and cause bloody digestions or stools."

WATER IN CONSUMPTION.

Water also is a drink that conduceth above all things to cure consumptive people, for the digestion being weakened, is the cause of producing a hot fretting nourishment, which is injurious to the tender substance of the lungs, and which constringes and stops up the lymphatic vessels through which the nourishment is to pass to all the parts; so that by degrees the body, for want of due supplies, consumes: which obstructions, and that acrimony which causeth them, will be opened and sweetened by the plentiful use of water, if taken before the lungs become ulcerous. Which cure of consumptions by water is recommended in the writings of Dr. Couch, who, in his "Praxis Catholica," tells us, that he knew a man cured very soon by drinking pure water. And it is said by another, that some have been cured of consumptions by drinking no other drink but water, avoiding all malt liquors and sharp wines: for wine or any other strong liquor is pernicious in this distemper, whose original is affirmed by Dr. Coward to be always in the stomach.

[But real consumption, in its advanced stages, is seldom cured by any means whatever. Water is the best remedy to palliate, but a cure can very seldom happen.]

HOT FLUSHES AND ERUPTIONS.

Some there are who are much troubled with flushing heat in the face, and others with a heat in the back; in both which cases, water used as a common drink is the best remedy, with a spare, cooling diet. And it is also excellent for such as have red blotches in their faces, which proceeds from a hot fretting blood, which, by water-drinking and a moderate diet, will be kept under. For, as Dr. Duncan, before quoted, doth affirm, those who keep their blood cool and clean are never troubled with breakings-out, like many others, who may be known to be drinkers of hot drinks, and use a hot full diet, by their faces being full of blotches.

COLIC.

Water is also commended by the learned for the colic; thus Riverius affirms, that in the colic large drinking of water hath been found to be an excellent remedy. And it is said by Fortis, that when he practiced at Venice, he often gave cold water in the colic with good success. With whom an English physician, Dr. Wainwright, in his Mechanical Account of the Six Non-naturals, concurs; for he saith, that water-drinkers are never troubled with the colic, and that many thereby have been cured when all other remedies failed.

[Professor Elliotson, of London, in "Principles and Practice of Medicine," says of this disease, "When every thing else has failed, I have known this affection of the bowels overcome, by taking the patient out of bed, and dashing two or three pails of cold water upon the abdomen."

Cold water suitably employed, is always favorable in relieving spasms of whatever kind. A person with the real spasmodic colic, could hardly be injured by water, however vigorous the application.]

SMALL-POX.

And in the small-pox, water hath also been proved to be an excellent drink. Salmon, in his Synopsis Medicine, saith, that in this distemper you may safely give the sick fair water, of which, says he, they may drink liberally to quench thirst; the want of which plenty of drink hath been the death of many a patient. Which opinion of his was right, as by experience I have found in two of my own children when sick of this distemper, to whom, after I had given a gentle vomit of emetic tartar, I gave no other drink but water, and they both recovered safely, and were not in the least light-headed, as two others before were in the same distemper, when treated otherwise. And I remember that one Dr. Betts being consulted in a case where the eruption did not come out kindly, did order two quarts of cold water to be drank as soon as could be; upon which they came out according to expectation, and the party did well.

[Dr. Baynard (1706) gives the following facts concerning the treatment of small-pox: Dr. Yarborough told me that his kinsman, Sir Thomas Yarborough, sent him a letter from Rome, wherein he gave him an account of a footman of his, who, when delirious in the small-pox, got from his bed, and in his shirt ran into a grotto of a cardinal's where there was water, in which he plunged himself, but was presently got out; the small-pox seemed to be sunk and struck in, but upon his going to bed they came out very kindly, and he safely recovered.

But my worthy and learned friend, Dr. Cole, showed me an account from an apothecary in Worcestershire, whose name (I think) was Mr. Matthews; the substance of which was, that a young man, delirious in the small-pox, when his nurse was asleep, jumped out of bed, ran down stairs, and went into a pond. The noise awakened the nurse, who followed with an outcry, which outcry raised the posse of the family, who surrounded the pond; but he parlied with them, and told them that if any body came in he would certainly drown them, and that he would come out when he saw his own time; and accordingly did so, and walked up stairs, and sat in his wet shirt, upon a chest by the bed-side; in which posture Mr. Matthews found him when he came into the chamber. Note here, that the apothecary lived three or four miles from the place, and he was in the water and on the chest all the while in his wet shirt that the messenger was gone for him. This apothecary, Mr. Matthews (for so I take his name), asked him how he did? He answered pretty well. He asked him if he would have a clean shirt, and go into bed? He said by-and-by he would; which accordingly he did. When in bed, he asked the apothecary if he had nothing good in his pocket, for he was a little faintish? He said that he had a cordial, of which he drank a good draught, so went to sleep, and awaked very well, and in a little time recovered. Now, as Dr. Cole observed very well, a man, quoth he, would not advise his patients in such a case to go into cold water, though this man escaped without injury; but it gives a good occasion to reflect on the many mischiefs that attend the small-pox in the hot regimen, since such extravagant and intense cold does so little or no harm.

Dr. Dover, of Bristol, told me of a vintner's drawer in Oxford, who in the small-pox went into a great tub of water, and there sat at least two hours, and yet the fellow recovered, and did well.

A gentleman, delirious in the small-pox, ran in his shirt, in the snow, at least a mile, and knocked them up in the house where he went, they being all in bed; the small-pox sunk, yet by the benefit of a looseness he recovered.

I remember about two years since, a learned gentleman, a divine, told me, that in the country where he was beneficed, in a small town not far from him, many died of a malignant small-pox. A certain boy, a farmer's son, was seized with a pain in his head and back, vomited, was feverish, etc., and had all the symptoms of the small-pox. This youth had promised some of his comrades to go a swimming with them that day, which notwithstanding his illness, he was resolved to do, and did so, but never heard more of his small-pox. Within three or four days, the father was seized just as the son was, and he was resolved to take Jack's remedy; his wife dissuaded him from it, but he was resolved upon it, and did immerge in cold water, and was after it very well. The worthy gentleman that told me this story, promised to give me it in writing, with the persons names and place; but I neglecting of it, he went out of town in two or three days, so I lost the opportunity of being better informed.

Mr. Lambert, brother to my worthy friend, Mr. Edmond Lambert, of Boyton, in the county of Wilts, told me, that when he was at school in Dorsetshire, at least thirty or more of the boys, one after another, fell sick of the small-pox, and that the nurse gave them nothing else but milk and apples in the whole course, and they all recovered. There was but one dissenting boy from that method, who, by command from his parents, went another course, and he had like to have died; nay, with very great difficulty they saved his life.]

BURNING FEVERS.

It is also certain, that in what we call burning fevers, water is found to be a safe and effectual remedy. It is said by Dr. Primrose, in his Popular Errors, that many great physicians have commended the drinking cold water in diseases, and they attribute to it the chief place in fevers, where the sick must drink largely; for thus taken, it will quench all heat (page 374). And Galen is said by an English author, to reprove Crastistratus for denying cold water in burning fevers; and says, that this is a remedy for any fever, provided it be drank in great abundance. With which opinion I find Dr. Oliver to agree, who, in his Essay on Fevers, says, that in fevers we must drink oftener than thirst calls for it, and such draughts as are plentiful; and the drink he prescribes, is either cold water or barley-water. Dr. Wainwright affirms also, that water is proper in fevers, and that the ancients gave as much of it as the patient could drink. And by another it is said, that if you give the patient nothing but water for three days, that in the third day the fever will be cured generally; but if it is not, give for food a little barley broth, and the fever will not exceed the seventh day. And by another we are informed, how one in a fever, that was past hope, being forbidden to drink water, which he greatly desired, did find means, in the absence of his nurse, to get a large pot-full, which he drank off, and lay down again, being well cooled, after which he fell into a sweat, and so was cured. And I find that Dr. Cook, of Warwick, in his book of Observations on English Bodies, does prescribe, for the cure of fevers, first a vomit, and afterward as much cold water as the patient can drink; and he saith, that if he sweat upon it, the sweat must be continued as long as can be. And it is said by another, that it is an excellent remedy in fevers, to drink a quart of hot water, and sweat upon it, being covered warm. There is also one Dr. Quinton, who, in his book of Observations, writes, that to one in a malignant fever, whose pulse was so low it could scarcely be felt, there were three quarts of water given at several draughts, to make him vomit; but it did not operate that way, yet the event was this: that it did refresh him, much raised his pulse, brought him into a breathing sweat, and passed off by urine; which lowness of the pulse my own experience hath often found to be raised by drinking water plentifully. And I know a woman, who, though she in a fever had the advice of two doctors, yet became distracted. I bid the nurse give her a pint of cold water, which she drank up, and in three or four minutes came to her right senses; and desiring to drink more, she recovered. And I have observed, that when, in fevers, the patient can relish no other drink, yet water is always drank with pleasure, as it will always be after eating sweet things, that spoil the relish of other drinks, which is one excellence peculiar to water, and shows it to be most agreeable to the nature of mankind, though now so much slighted. And besides this, it is a drink that will not turn sour in the stomach as all fermented drinks will do, to the increase of distempers already begun there.

[Dr. Baynard, that singular writer, gives a case thus:

"A Turk (a servant to a gentleman), falling sick of a fever, some one of the tribe of treacle-conners being called in, whether apothecary or physician, I can't tell, but (according to custom), what between blister and bolus, they soon made him mad. A countryman of his, that came to visit him, seeing him in the broiling condition, said nothing, but in the night-time, by some confederate help, got him down to the Thames-side, and soundly ducked him. The fellow came home sensible, and went to bed; and the next day he was perfectly well. This story was attested to by two or three gentlemen of undoubted integrity and worth; and I doubt it not, but believe it from the greater probability; for I'll hold ten to one on the Thames-side against treacle, snake-root, and all that hot regimen which inflames and exalts the blood, breaks its globules, and destroys the man. And then, forsooth, the doctor sneaks away like a dog that has lost his tail, and cries, it was a pestilential, malignant fever, that nobody could cure; and to show his care of the remainder, bids them open the windows, air the bed-clothes, and perfume the rooms for fear of infection; and if he be of the right whining, canting, prick-eared stamp, concludes, as they do at Tyburn, with a mournful ditty, a psalm, or a preservative prayer for the rest of the family. So exit Prig, with his starched, formal chops, ebony cane, fringed gloves, etc." Thus much for Dr. Baynard and his criticisms on doctors.]

GOUT.

And as for the gout, which Dr. Harris saith, in his anti-empiric, is gotten either by high feeding, or drinking much wine, or other strong drink, it may be cured, as that author doth affirm, by a very spare diet, and drinking water; according to what is said also by Sir Theodore Maybern, who, in his medicinal counsels, adviseth to leave off all strong drinks in this disease, and drink only water: and Van Heydon saith also, in his treatise of "Help for the Rich and Poor," that there not any greater remedy for the gout than drinking water, not only by young, but old men; many of whom, he saith, have drank cold water for many weeks, which hath succeeded so well, though they were far gone in years, that they found great ease thereby, without that offence to the stomach, or hindrance of digestion which some did seem to fear. And he also commends the large drinking of water in the sciatica, or hip-gout, he having often cured this distemper by this means, in less time than could reasonably be expected; and the same myself have found to be effectual in a pain in the shoulder, which had continued very bad for three months. For, being taken with a fever, I drank in one day about four quarts of water, which, though it did not make me sweat, because I lay not in my bed, yet it cured me so that I slept well that night; and in the morning when I rose, I did find that the pain in my shoulder was not felt, neither did it ever return. And the same success I have had in the pains of other parts, whereby I judge, that in all pains whatever, the drinking of water is proper, as well as in the gout; and accordingly I find cold water advised to be drank largely for the cure of the headache from hard drinking, that pain proceeding from the same cause the gout does, namely, from heat, as all pains do that are not from bruises.

INFLAMMATORY DISEASES.

It is said also by Dr. Wainwright, that in the itch, scurvy, leprosy, and in all hot inflammatory distempers, such as pleurisies, rheumatisms, and St. Anthony's fire, water is a proper remedy; but he adviseth to drink it hot in some cases, as doubtless it ought to be done in pleurisies. He also saith, that water is proper in headaches, catarrhs, vapors, falling sickness, dullness of sight, melancholy, shortness of breath, scurvy in the mouth, and windiness in the stomach: and for wind in the stomach, I by long experience have found it the best remedy, who, in the former part of my life, through a disorderly diet, and drinking strong drink like others, was never free from windy belchings, and sometimes very sickish qualms after meals; from which at length I was delivered, by drinking only water at meals, so that for above forty years I have been seldom troubled; and if I find myself troubled, a pint or more of cold water in less than half an hour will set me free, by drinking of it.

HARD DRINKING.

And that water is the best remedy for the mischiefs that come by hard drinking, experience teacheth; there being nothing that so effectually frees from those nauseating and retching qualms the next morning, as the drinking of a pint or more of fair water; which effectually allays the inflammation of the bowels, occasioned by strong or hot drink, which spoils the strength of the stomach, as it doth the strength of all other parts; nothing being a greater enemy to the vigor of the nerves and sinews, since by much drinking men make themselves unable to stand or go: which effect would never follow, if liquors that abound with spirits were strengthening; and if they were strengthening, the fibres of the stomach would not be so weakened after drinking strong drinks, as to make men sick; which sickness will soon be recovered by the drinking cold water, this being also the best remedy, if taken largely, for that heat of urine which is often occasioned by hard drinking.

COLDS.

In colds, water is the best of all drinks to prevent floods of rheum from the nose and mouth, as my long experience testifies, and the drinking therefore will prevent coughs, for a cough will seldom succeed a cold, if water is used from the first as a common drink; and if through neglect, a cough should become troublesome, the use of water, avoiding all wine or strong drink, will contribute much to the cure. Some order the water to be drank warm, but others say that the drinking it cold vastly excels the using it hot in a cough. It is said by Van Heydon, that some may think it strange to advise water in such diseases, which most do account to proceed from crudity or indigestion; but he says, that in any disease where the case is dangerous, the use of water is the only friend to nature; cold water being a preventer rather than a cause of crudity, since by all experience, it is proved to be a promoter of a good digestion: and at this time, I know a woman seventy-eight years of age, who, for this ten years past, hath had a great cough, and spit much tough phlegm, that this present winter, 1722, hath been persuaded to leave off all strong and small fermemted liquor, and drink only water at meals, and sometimes a dish or two of tea, and hath found herself much less subject to cough than before, and scarce coughs at all in bed, though subject before to cough very much in the night; she also drinks at bed-time half a pint of cold water, and the same quantity first in the morning, and finds herself more comforted by it at so great an age, than wine hath at any time afforded.

STRONG DRINKS HURTFUL TO CHILDREN.

It is generally the opinion of most physicians, that wine and strong drinks are not proper for children, and that the smaller and cooler their drink is, the better it will be with them; and that nothing conduceth more to the health of children than drinking water, which will prevent the foundation of those diseases that are caused in many by strong drink, and do show themselves in their more advanced age, wherein many also do suffer much by the mother's ill custom of making them gluttons, by constantly cramming their stomachs with food, many being thereby destroyed among the children of the rich before they come to years of maturity; when the children of poor country people, who fare hard, stand their ground till full grown. For fewer children die in the country than in great cities, where luxury in diet doth more abound which is one reason why so few housekeepers in London were born in it, the great supply of inhabitants being from the country, children being brought up more hardy there than in London, where great numbers are killed by over-pleasing their palates. Which mischief would be in a great measure prevented by their being accustomed to eat less and drink water; which, by experience, is found to make young children free from that frowardness which is commonly caused by a sharp and hot, or feverish blood, which engendereth wind and causeth pain and gripes. For there is no pain but is the consequence of heat, or inward as well as outward inflammations.

To what hath been said, may be added this consideration, that when the best physicians are baffled by some diseases, they advise their patients to use the water of some mineral spring; tacitly acknowledging thereby, that all their prescriptions may be excelled by water. They pretend, indeed, to ascribe its effects to some minerals with which the waters are tinctured. But Dr. Baynard, in page 438 of Sir John Floyer's Cold Bathing, tells of a certain person who used to frequent Tunbridge, by which he found much benefit; but being hindered from going thither one season, did drink the same quantity of water taken from the pump of a spring in his own yard, which did him as much service; whereupon he wrote thus on his pump:

"The steel is a cheat;
'Tis water does the feat."

And, indeed, if we consider how many diseases and pains proceed from a sizy thick blood, which cannot pass as it ought to do through the finest pipes that convey the blood to the parts, pure water, without minerals, drank to the quantity of a quart or three pints in a morning, will attenuate or thin the blood sufficiently—nothing, as Boerhaave affirms, being a greater diluter of thick blood, than warm water drank in great quantity; which to thin the blood may be best, though to strengthen the stomach it is best drank cold; having the same

4*

effect inwardly, in some cases, as cold bathing hath outwardly; its use outwardly being also great.

BURNS AND SCALDS.

Water, I have found by long experience, to be of excellent use in burns and scalds; for in all burns and scalds that are slight, if the part is plunged immediately into cold water, the colder the better, the pain will instantly be taken off; and it will fetch out the fire, if continued so long as will be required to do it by any other remedy. And if the burn be so considerable that other remedies must be applied, none of which will take off the smart of themselves in less than two or three hours, yet if you apply cold water presently after other applications are made to the part, the pain will immediately cease, till the remedy becomes effectual; so that the ease water will give in such cases, makes it of good use. Which remedy, as it hath not been discovered till now, appears to transcend all other remedies in this case; because, in a moment the great smart will be eased, if the water is cold, and will be felt no more if the part afflicted be kept immersed in it till the fire is extinguished, either by the water, or the medicine applied. Besides, it is a remedy every where ready at hand, which cannot be said of any other; which generally requires so much time to get it ready, that much pain will be endured, if blisters do not arise, which do much increase the trouble. If the part burnt or scalded cannot be dipped in water, you may apply water to it with double linen cloths dipped therein, and new dipped as they grow warm; by which means I have cured burns and scalds in the face without blistering, when applied immediately before blisters did arise.

[In the Water-Cure Journal of July 1st, 1846, we published the following cases, illustrative of the truly wonderful effects of water in the treatment of scalds and burns:

"A few weeks since we were sent for in great haste, to visit the infant child of Mrs. Campbell, a sempstress of this city, whose case of child-birth was some time since given in the Journal. The message was, that the child was very severely scalded. We hastened to the woman's residence, and there learned the following particulars: The little fellow (being ten months old, and a cold-water child, so called) was, as usual, running about the room, playfully, when he drew down upon himself, from a bench, or low table, a large pitcher full of hot water. The fluid passed upon his neck, shoulder, down the arm, upon the side, abdomen, over about one third of the back, and upon one foot. The whole extent of these parts was scalded, and in places blisters rose, apparently as thick as one's finger. In consequence of the wonderful effects of water which the mother had herself experienced before the birth of her infant, as well as at that time and subsequently, and what she had witnessed in rearing, thus far, the child—he never having had an hour's sickness from the first, or taken a single particle of medicine—she had very naturally the greatest confidence in the new treatment. She preferred, in fact, rather to treat the case herself, than have a physician of the ordinary practice—such a one having been called, through mistake of the messenger, and arriving very soon after the accident. The mother said there was a mistake—he was not the right doctor; so he took a look at the little patient, well wrapped up in a wet sheet (it being, no doubt, the first time he had ever witnessed the 'bug-bear' application), and then turned upon his heel and left.

"Immediately after the accident, the little sufferer began to collapse, as the term is; he grew pale and cold, and had a severe chill. The mother instantly wrapped him in a folded wet sheet; but his appearing to be cold, led her quickly to place about him an abundance of warm blankets, outside the sheet. It was nòt long before what is called, in such cases, reaction, began to take place; the circulation and heat increased, and, at the same time, the pain. All these symptoms were in themselves favorable, but demanded, at the same time, the most prompt treatment. The mother had already, before we arrived, very properly commenced cooling the affected parts, by frequently changing the wet cloths. We directed her to have the child held over a tub of water, and to pour cold water constantly upon the cloths, these remaining upon the scalded parts, and to continue this process as long as the pain remained. She kept on thus cooling the scalded surface, until her suffering child ceased his piteous moaning and went to sleep. This must have taken place between two and three hours after the accident. He slept awhile, and awoke apparently as bright as usual. Still, so much of the surface was either blistered or abraded, that he could scarcely move without causing much distress. Those parts were directed to be kept constantly covered with fine linen cloths, wet, and these to be covered with dry ones, so that the system might not become too much chilled. The child was to have as much water as he chose to drink, to be fed very sparingly, and the windows were to be left open both night and day, for the admission of fresh air. The mother followed the directions faithfully, and, in a very short time, the parts were perfectly healed. During the first afternoon, every trace of the inflammation, where the surface was not actually destroyed, was removed. The fire, as some would say, was completely drawn out.

"This cure may be properly divided into two more prominent parts: first, the cooling means used until the abnormal heat was removed; and secondly, the soothing or poultice effect of the moist applications that were continued until the healing of the parts was fully accomplished. What is there that will at all compare with the pure element in causing animal as well as vegetable growth? Throughout all nature, in both vegetable and animal bodies, water is the great fluid through which the vital processes are carried on.

"We think the medical friend who saw this case, in connection with us, will agree that burns of apparently not more than one third the severity of this, frequently cause death in a few hours."

We published also, in the same number, the following facts from an Ohio paper, which came to us on authority that may be fully relied on as being correct. The narrator gives them as follows:

"In the 12th month of 1843, as I was going to Piqua, I met a wagon with a sick man in it, lying upon a bed. He seemed to be traveling in much pain. I inquired the cause of his suffering, and was told that he was scalded by the bursting of steam works in a tan-yard near Piqua, about fourteen days before; that he was an apprentice to Mr. McTurnahan, a tanner, and that McTurnahan was also scalded, with two of his sons. But the old man, who was the most scalded of any, jumped immediately into the pool, which was slightly frozen over, and came out entirely well.

"This tale appeared so marvelous, that I concluded to call at the residence of McTurnahan, and make further inquiries. I did so; and was informed by the old man, that he, his two sons, and apprentice, were standing near the boiler of heating water when it burst. He stood in such a position as to take the strongest current of water and steam. This is the only evidence he has that he was scalded as the others, for he jumped immediately into the pool, and directed the boys to follow him. On coming out, and feeling the pain continue, he went in again. The skin pealed off a little from the lower part of his arms, and a little from his breast. This was all the mark he had upon him, and it had not hindered him from his work at all. He supposes he was not in the water more than five minutes.

"His oldest son came to the brink of the pool, and stepped in about half way up to his knees. He then stopped to unbutton his clothes, and see how badly he was hurt. Finding the skin peel off with his clothes, as he took them down, he concluded to go into the house and send for the doctor. It was within three or four days of six months before he was able to go about again. But so far as he went into the pool, there was no mark of hot water upon him. The youngest son was scalded only upon his legs. He went immediately into the pool, as his father had directed. The only mark left upon him was a small sore on one of his heels.

"The apprentice went into the house, and was doctored according to custom. It was two weeks before he could be taken home upon a bed, and four months before he could go about.

"I have called several times at McTurnahan's, once in company with Samuel Jay and Walter D. Jay, members of the society of Friends, who lived in Miami county. The statement he makes is uniform, and I think may be relied upon.

"Thine, etc., AUGUSTUS WATTLES."

"MERCER Co., O., 5th month, 1st, 1846."

To those who have never witnessed the effects of cold water in scalds or burns, statements like the above appear like mere idle fiction; but those who have witnessed such effects, recognize, at once, upon the face of such narrations, their truth.]

ULCERS.

I once knew a large ulcer in the foot, made by the running of melted brass into the shoe, that was kept in hand by a surgeon nine weeks, without any probability of healing, because of the great inflammation that attended it; but the party being a lover of angling, was persuaded to go with some others to Hackney river. Some of them went bare-legged into the water, to come at a certain hole where much fish was sometimes found. The sport was so good that the lame man, having pulled off his stockings and plasters, went in also, where he staid above two hours, and, coming out again, he found the ulcer, which appeared very red and angry when he went in, did look pale. He put on his dressings and came home, and in less than a fortnight his ulcer healed up; which doubtless was occasioned by the abating of the inflammation by the coldness of the water. And I have had an account also from an acquaintance, that was surgeon to a merchant ship, that their gunner, at a time when the captain treated some friends on board, going to charge a gun that just before had been fired off, the cartridge he was ramming down took fire, whereby he was blown into the water, and had some of his fingers torn off, and it was an hour before a boat could be got to take him up. But they found that the coldness of the water had almost stopped the bleeding, and the cure was effected so speedily, that other surgeons wondered at it; which he imputed to the water, which kept back the humors, by its coldness, from flowing to the part at the first; so that there was no impediment from inflammation to hinder healing; for the chief impediment to healing is inflammation, in wounds or ulcers.

SPRAINS.

And as for strains and sprains in the joints, cold water affords the best and most speedy remedy, as Van Heydon affirms; who saith, that by bathing in cold water all harm so received may, by this remedy, be cured more safely and more speedily than by any other, without loss of time, cost, or trouble; for no more is to be done, as I have often found, than, as soon as can be, to put the part into a vessel of cold water for about two hours, which will prevent all swelling and pain, by repelling or keeping back the humors that otherwise would flow to the part. And if it should be the shoulder, or any other part, which is so hurt, that cannot well be immersed in water after this manner, water may be applied, by dipping towels folded up into it, and laying them to the part, as is done, in effect, to the wrenched joints of horses, about which, if you wind oftentimes a thick rope made of hay, and then cast upon it divers times a pail of cold water, the wrench will be cured; which experiment is now commonly practiced by those concerned about horses.

WEAKNESS IN THE JOINTS.

Bathing in cold water hath also been found to be a good remedy to strengthen weakness in the joints, as Sir John Floyer, in his Treatise of Cold Bathing, hath shown; and which by experience I found to be true in a certain woman, who complained of great weakness and pain in her ankles. I advised her to dip the part in cold water every morning for a quarter of an hour, and do the same at night; and in about twenty days she became as strong in that part as she was in the other. And Sir John tells us of a boy who could not stand, his limbs were so weak, that by bathing in cold water perfectly recovered his strength in a little time.

PAIN IN THE HEAD.

Great pain in the head hath been also cured by this means; for we are told by Van Heydon, that one Sir Toby Matthews had for twenty years been troubled with great pain in one side of the head, and a great defluxion of rheum from his nose; but he at last was cured, by applying cold water to the part every day for about a quarter of an hour; upon reading of which, I tried the experiment upon myself, who for a long time had been troubled with the running of much clear water from my nose, with great spitting of thin rheum; for I let a water-cock run upon the mould of my head every morning, by which, in about six weeks' time, I was eased of my trouble. And since that I had a credible information of a certain servant-maid, who was afflicted greatly with a rheumatism, and an intolerable pain in the head, who, being put into St. Thomas's Hospital, her nurse was ordered by the doctor to apply to her head towels four times double, dipped in cold water, changing them as they became warm, which she was to continue doing four or five hours; in which time she was freed from that pain in the head, and was afterward cured of the rheumatism by other means.

WANT OF SLEEP IN FEVERS.

The want of sleep in fevers may be cured likewise by the application of cold water. For to a near relation in a fever, who could not sleep for three days and three nights, I ordered a towel to be several times folded up, and then to be dipped in water, and a little wrung out, and so laid upon her forehead, and to be new dipped as it grew hot; which in about two hours' time so cooled her head, that she fell into a sleep, and continued in it five hours. And I ordered the same to be done the next night, with the same success. And we find that Dr. Cockburn, in his Treatise of Sea Diseases, did order, for the want of sleep in fevers, to dip a towel, four times doubled, in oxycrat, which is six parts water and one part vinegar, to be bound about the head and temples; which, he saith, will cause sleep with wonderful success. But cold water only will have the same effect, as I often have proved.

SWOONINGS.

And that the use of cold water in swoonings is of great effect, common experience teacheth ; for, if a dish or cup of cold water is thrown strongly upon the face, the person in an instant will recover, though for a time he seemeth dead, and perhaps might not have recovered in some cases, if cold water had not been so applied; such faintings being sometimes deadly, which proceed from poisonous vapors ascending up to the brain from a foul stomach; for such effects there are, as I have found by experience, who in my young days did swoon away twice; at both which times I was sensible of a collection of wind in my stomach, from whence I plainly felt a fume or vapor ascend to my head, that in an instant deprived me of all sense. But being both times in the company of a person who had seen the thing tried, he dashed some cold water against my face, which I remember made me start, as if I had been suddenly awaked. And I am apt to think that some die in such a fit, when none are near to help them ; and especially when so taken in their sleep, which I believe none need fear who live temperately, or that eat no suppers ; none who have refrained from suppers having been ever found to die in sleep.

BLEEDINGS AT THE NOSE.

Dangerous bleedings at the nose have also been cured with cold water largely drank, syringing cold water up their nostrils, and applying towels round their necks dipped in cold water, changing them as they grow warm ; for it is said by a good writer, that this will so cool the heat of the blood, and by the coldness of the water syringed up the nose, so contract the mouths of the veins which bleed, that it will put a stop to the bleeding. Such bleedings have also been stopped by dashing cold water often into the face, as a French writer hath affirmed, whose name was Flamand; and the same, also, is affirmed by Cook, in his Marrow of Surgery.

SMALL CUTS.

Cold water is an absolute cure for all small cuts in the fingers, or other parts; for if, when cut, you close the cut up with the thumb of your other hand, keeping it so closed for a quarter or half an hour, this will infallibly stop the bleeding; after which, if you double up a linen rag five or six times, dip it in cold water, and apply it to the part, binding it on, this, by preventing inflammation and a flux of humors, will give nature time soon to heal it without any other application, as is seen in the common practice of surgeons when they let a man bleed; for all the application they make to the vein so cut, is a pledget of linen dipped in cold water, and bound on with a fillet; for all wounds without loss of substance will heal of themselves, if inflammation be prevented, and the lips of the wound are kept close together.

BITINGS OF A MAD DOG.

We also are told by Van Heydon, that in his time some were of an opinion, that a person bit by a mad dog might be preserved from that symptom called the fear of water, which generally follows, and proves so mortal, by applying cold water to the place bitten. And this, he says, they conceive to be no unlikely thing, if there is any credit to be given to what Cornelius Celsus writes, who saith, that the only remedy in this case is to throw the party who is in this condition, or hath the fear of water upon him, into a pond or river, and when plunged over head and ears, to keep him in the water till filled with it, whether he will or no; and by this means both his thirst and dread of water will be cured. For if this immersion be of use when the party is so far gone, why should it not be of greater force in preserving from it, if speedily applied and repeated? Now, though this is mentioned by him as a probable opinion, yet experience in our days shows, that the plunging the patient into the salt water either of the river Thames about Gravesend, or in the salt springs in Cheshire, is the best means to prevent any evil succeeding the bite of a mad dog. They must indeed be dipped so often as to be almost drowned before the danger is over. But it is a question whether the saltness of the water contributes any thing to this cure, since Boerhaave, the present professor at Leyden, affirms, that when men bitten by a mad dog are arrived to the fear of water, called an hydrophobia, they may be cured by blinding the patient's eyes, and throwing of him into a pond of water often, till he seems not to be afraid of it, or but very little, and then force him to drink large quantities.

FALLING SICKNESS.

And we are told by Dr. Edward Browne, that a person troubled with the falling sickness, by happening to fall into a cold spring (I suppose it was in the time of his fit), was freed from his distemper all his life after;

and he saith there is no need of preparing the body for it in this, as in some other cases. But the patient, when plunged into a cold bath, ought to continue in the bath each time about three or four minutes; for in plunging over head and ears at his first entrance into a cold bath, the brain will be so sensibly affected, as to be relieved from the distemper, which is a kind of convulsion proceeding from an inflammation, or some other cause: but we want more experiments to confirm this notion; which notion may be worth noting, that the thing may be tried in others, to see whether it will succeed as it did in this person. For it is said by the ingenious Dr. Pitcairn, a Scotchman, some time professor at Leyden, that there is no such thing as the art of curing, but only the practice—that remedies were found out by chance (p. 264 of his works); for when remedies thus happen to be discovered, and prove often to be effectual, the remembering that remedy, to apply it in a like case in practice, brings reputation to the prescriber; but if it fails, some other experiment must be tried, which, were physic an art, need not be done, because the rules of art are certain, and men depend upon them as such.

MADNESS AND MELANCHOLY.

It is also said by the same Dr. Browne, that madness and melancholy, with all their retinue, may find better effects from the use of bathing in cold water, than from other violent methods, with which people so afflicted are now treated; for, says he, that which will make a drunken man sober in a minute, will certainly go a great way toward the cure of a madman in a month. Now it is most certain, to my own knowledge, that if a drunken man be plunged over head and ears in cold water, he will come out of it perfectly sober. And some I have known, that in such cases have been recovered by barely washing their heads in cold water. Which fore-mentioned opinion of Dr. Browne is confirmed by the practice of Dr. Blair, who, in a letter to Dr. Baynard, declares, that he cured a man raving mad, who being bound in a cart, stripped of his clothes, and blindfolded, that the surprise might be the greater, he on a sudden had a great fall of water let down upon him from the height of twenty feet, under which he continued so long as his strength would permit; and after his return home, he fell into a sleep, and slept twenty-nine hours, and awakened in as quiet a state of mind as ever, and so had continued to the time of writing that letter, which was twelve months. Distraction also in fevers, of which there are divers instances in the History of Cold Baths, has been cured by being plunged in cold water.

Which relation seems to make that a more probable truth, which was related in a letter from Sir John Floyer to Dr. Browne, and printed by that doctor; wherein it is said, that, in Normandy, they immerse fools, or dip them in cold water, to cure them: a hot brain being the cause, perhaps, of several disorders in the understanding, and is in great part found to be true, in the ridiculous behavior of some drunken men, which, when their heads are become cool, abhor what they before did do or say. Now if such dipping would cure fools among us, great numbers might be made more happy than they are by being so dipped.

KING'S EVIL.

Dr. Browne, in his Discourse of Cold Baths, affirms likewise, that to bathe in cold water, hath been found to be the quickest, safest, and pleasantest cure for the king's evil; and he tells us (in p. 85) of a Yorkshire gentleman, who was grievously afflicted with this distemper, having great ulcers in the glands of his neck, which were so much inflamed as to bring him very low; but being advised by Dr. Baynard to bathe in the cold bath, he in a month's time was perfectly cured, his ulcers being healed up, contrary to the opinion of the most learned physicians.

JAUNDICE.

We also find mention, in the description of the Scottish islands, of an odd remedy, commonly made use of there for the cure of the jaundice; which is this: They strip the party naked, lay him upon the ground, on his belly, and pour, unawares, upon his back a pail of cold water.

PAINFUL JOINTS.

And also pains in the joints, as Dr. Curtis tells us, will be cured, by holding the part under the stream of a pump or cock; and fomenting with cold water is commended, as good to assuage hot swellings.

INFLAMED EYES.

And I know a person who had often been subject to blood-shot or inflamed eyes, who afterward, upon the beginning of the same distemper, took, by advice, a ball of linen rags, dipped them in cold water, and applied them to the part, cooling them by new dipping as oft as they grew hot: which application was continued three hours, in which time the humor was so repelled, as to be troublesome no more; for the party, to my knowledge, hath had no sign of that distemper since, though the same had been very troublesome many times before.

COLD WATER FOR THE EYES.

It is also advised, by Dr. Gideon Harvey, to wash the eyes well, twice a day in cold water, as the best remedy to prevent defluxions on them, and preserve the eyesight, which it greatly comforts. And this I have found true for many years, my eyes being often apt to be dim and stiff, so that I could scarce open my eye-lids; which, upon washing for a minute with fair water, hath been felt no more for a good while after. Besides which benefit to the eyes, authors say it is also good to preserve the memory, if the whole forehead be washed twice a day; which also is a certain cure for itching in the eyes, as authors tell us. And, indeed, washing with water will free mankind from a troublesome itching in any other part of the body, let it be never so private, as Cook, in his Observations on English Bodies, doth expressly declare from experience.

CALLOSITIES OF THE FEET.

Some people are troubled with a callosity, or hardness of the bottoms of their feet, which is so troublesome, as to be a hindrance to their easy walking; for which a cure is prescribed by Dr. Cook, that is, to soak them well in warm water, till the hardness is softened, and then scrape it off with the edge of a knife: and if the feet burn with any unnatural heat, the bathing often in hot water will cool them, by giving vent to what offends. [But cold water is the better remedy.]

SCURVY.

And the plentiful drinking of water is commended in the scurvy, whether hot or cold, by Dr. Pitcairn, to dissolve the scorbutic salts, and carry them out by urine, whether they are acids or alkalies; and myself having formerly been extremely troubled with the scurvy, which often made me faint and weak, and my pulse so low as scarcely to be felt, did find at last that the pulse would infallibly rise upon drinking a pint or more of cold water, and in a little time I should again become brisk and strong: for I have often observed, that upon a disorder of the stomach, the strength of the bodily members soon would fail, and as easily be recovered when the disorder of the stomach was removed; yea, by long experience, I have found that nothing conduceth so much to bodily strength as a stomach in right order, which requires temperance and cooling diet to bring it into order, when distempered.

ASTHMA.

To what hath been already said, I will add an account, taken from a credible person, of a man in the parish of Shoreditch, who was desperately ill of an asthma, or shortness of breath, and deep consumption, for which he had tried many remedies to no purpose. At length he was advised by a physician, being poor, to drink no other drink but water, and eat no other food but water-gruel, without salt or sugar; which course of diet he continued for three months, finding himself at first to be somewhat better, and at the three months' end he was perfectly cured: but, for security sake, he continued in that diet a month longer, and grew strong and fat upon it. But his diet he had no mind to, till he was thoroughly hungry, and then he ate it with pleasure; in which, perhaps, consisted the best part of his cure, it being an advantage to health never to eat till hunger calls for food.

COUGH.

And I remember a young woman, a burnisher of silver, who had a desperate cough, for which she had taken many things of an apothecary to no purpose; at length the journeyman told her, his master said he could do no more; but, said the fellow, I would advise you every morning to wash behind your ears, and upon your temples, and on the mould of your head with cold water; which she told me she did, and was perfectly cured of her cough by that means.

DIFFICULTY IN MAKING WATER.

There are divers other cases wherein the use of water hath done much good. I knew an ancient practicer in physic, who told me, that in many difficulties of making water, he had advised the party to put his private member into water, as hot as he could endure it, which, in a minute, did cause him to make water; and that women have had the same benefit by sitting over hot water. And he often had advised them who were costive, and went to stool with great difficulty, to sit over a pot with hot water in it; which soon was attended with an easy dejection, or stool, the body drawing up the vapor, which did provoke expulsion of the excrements without much straining.

[Injections of water, cold, if the person is not extremely weak, are excellent in constipation. So, also, Priessnitz's wet girdle and the hip-bath. In strangury, cold water is far better than hot or warm; but the use of warm water is far better than none at all. Cold water, however, is the great thing. Putting the feet upon a cold floor, or in cold water, or holding the hands in cold water, are well known to cause a disposition to void urine. But the cold hip-bath, and the general ablutions in cold water, are the more effectual means.]

And it hath been observed, that froward children have been made much more quiet, by washing their lower parts every morning with water, to wash off the salts of their urine, which usually stick in the pores of the skin, and are fretful and uneasy, and nothing cures their soreness about those parts like it. Nor is there any thing more effectual to cure men, who are galled with riding, than to wash themselves well, when they go to bed, with cold water; and washing the bare breast every morning with cold water, will make those hardy who before were apt at every turn to take cold. To which I will add this, that Sir Theodore Maybern affirms, in his Medicinal Counsels, that, in most diseases of the head, there is nothing better than to bathe it with cold water, which, in a desperate pain in the ears, upon taking cold, I have found to be true; for the pain seemed to vanish upon applying to it about thirty minutes, a towel doubled up often, and wet in cold water; and though it returned again some hours after, yet ease was obtained the same way, and the cure perfected in four times doing: which cure of a pain gotten with cold, by a cold application, will not seem so strange, when we consider that in the northern countries, mortifications from cold are no ways to be cured but by applying cold snow.

In short, water when rightly made use of, doth appear from the accounts before mentioned, very effectual to prevent and cure many diseases, but more especially the inward use thereof; for, to use the words of the ingenious Dr. Curtis, in his Essay for the Preservation and Recovery of Health, the habitual use of water for common drink, preserves the native ferment of the stomach in due order, keeps the blood temperate, and helps to spin out the thread of life to the longest extent of nature; it makes the rest at night more quiet and refreshing, the reason and understanding more clear, the passions less disorderly; and in case of eating too much, a large draught of cold water vastly exceeds any other cordial to cause digestion, water being not so cold and lifeless, as many do imagine. Besides which commendation of it by this doctor, it is certainly a drink that will not ferment in the stomach, nor turn sour, as wine and strong malt drinks will do, to the hindering of a good digestion, which all acidity in the stomach certainly doth, when it abounds there; and is best corrected by weakening or making it less sour, by drinking good store of water, as the experience of above forty years' practice hath assured myself and many others. For though water is accounted a contemptible drink, yet by beginning to make use of it at about thirty years of age, before which I was

6

often out of order, and continuing the use of it ever since, drinking very little wine or strong drink, I have attained to the age of seventy-four years; when thousands, in the meantime, who delighted only in drinking strong beer, wine, and brandy, have not lived half so long; which makes good that saying in the Scriptures, that "wine is a mocker, and strong drink is raging, and he who is deceived thereby is not wise" (Prov. xx. 1), since it no ways contributes to long life; for it is certain that thousands in the world live as long who drink no strong drink, as any drinkers of it do. Some, indeed, from an extraordinary strength of nature, have been hard drinkers, and yet die old; but for one who does this, perhaps an hundred are destroyed by it before they come to half the time of life; and generally we shall find that very strong and healthy constitutions, at the long run, are ruined by riot and excess, there being no certain safety in any way of living, but that of temperance and moderation. Nature, in some, may a long time withstand the abuses offered to it, but at last it will yield to its enemies; and those who live the longest in an intemperate course, might, from the strength of their constitution, have lived much longer had they eat less, and used themselves to drink more water; which drink, as it is most friendly, and will preserve longest the life of a strong constitution, so it is absolutely necessary for those that are weak and sickly, and are naturally subject to the gout, the stone, shortness of breath, wind, ill-digestion, and such like.

WATER USEFUL IN VOMITING.

But the chief use of water in preserving of health, is by using of it as a vomit, as before was shown, which is an infallible and the most speedy remedy that ever was found out for any stomach-sickness or pain there; for to vomit with warm water will effectually remove it in one hour, and be a means to prevent great fits of sickness, and preserve the lives of many thousands to old age, by cleansing the stomach from that tough, slimy, or corrupt matter that offends, and is the cause of all mortal diseases; especially of an apoplexy, which though counted a disease of the head, yet hath its original from a foul stomach, which nothing doth so effectually cleanse as vomits: according to that of Dr. Curtis, who saith, that vomiting with warm water or carduus tea, is very beneficial to bring up that which fluctuates in the stomach, and that tough, ropy phlegm, which sticks fast to the wrinkles and folds of that bowel, and which purges do often pass over, and cannot remove. Which way of vomiting with warm water is ten times more easy and pleasant than that which is effected by the use of a nauseous tea made of carduus, which physicians do sometimes advise; and it is also such as can do no harm by violence, as other vomits made from antimony sometimes do, for want of drinking after each vomit a pint or more of water-gruel, or warm water, since you may stop when you please, by forbearing to drink more warm water, when you vomit with water.

And here it may not be amiss to relate what I some years ago discovered, in order to men's freeing themselves from sickness that may happen after eating; for being invited to dine at a certain table, where there were several good dishes of meat, I was over-persuaded to eat more than I should do, and in a little time after dinner found myself begin to be sick. I went out, and in a private place attempted to vomit, by tickling my throat with my finger, but could not vomit as I designed to do; only by this means I raised up two or three mouthfuls of thick, tough phlegm, upon which I found myself better, and my sick qualm went off. I took the hint it gave me, and have done the same several times since, and find that by getting up the phlegm, which, like yeast upon beer, works up to the mouth of the stomach, a man may free himself from some kinds of sickness after eating. And I remember it is an advice given by one Vaughan, in a book long since printed, entitled Directions for Health, for men who feed high, to put their finger in their throat when they rise in the morning, to make themselves puke, or avoid the phlegm which can be raised, as an excellent way to preserve health; and it is said also to be an absolute preservative from the gout.

GRIPINGS.

I will conclude with this note, that in such distempers, where water-drinking will be available for a cure, the same must not be drank sparingly, but plentifully, as (for instance) to ease the gripings in a looseness or flux; for if but a pint of water should be drank, ease would hardly succeed; but drinking in about an hour's time a quart or three pints, the sharpness and evil quality of the humor offending will be so far diluted or weakened, that immediate ease will follow. If the season be too cold to drink cold water, you may warm it a little upon the fire, or put a hot toast of bread into every pint; and the same is true in fevers, or in pains from gravel or the colic. A small quantity will not be effectual in these cases, for in the colic a quart is necessary, which ought to be carefully noted; and in a fever a little water will rather increase the burning, which large draughts, often drank, will soon take off. Rest, fasting, and drinking much water, after a vomit or two, is a course that never yet hath failed to cure fevers, by clearing the stomach of that sordid filthiness which causeth the distemper; for a happy issue will certainly follow such a course, if the fever is simple, and not complicated with such other distempers, which will resist all remedies; for in many cases nothing can prevent mortality, as is evident by the death of the best physicians themselves, and by the death of many who consulted with them for a cure, since many die under the hands of the most able doctors as well as quacks.

GRIEF AND FRIGHT.

I will add to what hath been said one experiment more that is very material; and that is, being very hypochondriacal, and of a melancholy temper, I have often been strangely dejected in mind, when under grief for some misfortunes, which sometimes have been so great as to threaten danger to life; in which fits of grief I always found the parts within my breast very uneasy, and sometimes continued long; but now I have found a good remedy, for upon drinking a pint or more of cold water, I find ease in two or three minutes, so that no grief seems to afflict. Which experience I discover for the sake of others in the same circumstances, being verily persuaded that the stomach sympathizeth with the mind, and this becomes the cause of that uneasy sensation and pain perceived there; for which, cold water I have found to be the best remedy in myself, and I believe others may find the same benefit, who will make use thereof upon the like occasion; and it gives also relief to people under frights.

VAPORS, OR HYSTERICS.

There is also another experiment that I have often seen of good effect; and that is, if persons subject to what is called vapors, or that are afflicted with fits, commonly called the fits of the mother, will but drink water when they find their fits approach, it will immediately yield relief. There is in this case a mealy julep prescribed by Dr. Bates, which is, to take a spoonfull of fine wheat flour, an ounce of fine sugar, and a pint of water, brew them together, and drink it off. This is pleasanter than water alone; but water of itself will be as effectual, or rather better, as hath been often proved upon persons in those fits.

HOW TO DISTINGUISH GOOD WATER.

Some persons may desire to know how to distinguish good from bad water; and the way to do this is by the taste and scent; for if it have no taste nor smell, being purely fresh, not salt, nor sweetish, nor ill-scented, it is good, provided it be pure and clear; of which kind is the common water used in London, when well settled, or in fair weather. As for those who are curious, and will be at the charge, they may procure the best water for drink by distillation, either in an alembic, or in a cold still used in drawing any cold water from herbs; for no earthy or metallic substance, nor any kind of salt, will rise in distillation; so that the water so distilled will be pure and admirable to drink when cold, and will keep as long from stinking as any of the cold distilled water in the apothecaries' shops, according to what Dr. Quincy hath affirmed about it in his dispensatory.

Those who have not the convenience of distillation, may boil it a little, as they do for tea; for then, when kept a while after it is cold, it will become more fine, by suffering any mixture contained in it to settle to the bottom of the vessel wherein it is contained, and that will render it still more pure. In short, all water that will make a good lather with soap, is wholesome to drink without boiling, and none else.

[Rain-water, when obtained pure, is excellent for both cooking and drinking. It can easily be filtered if need be; and every family may have it in abundance, at a comparatively small expense, in erecting cisterns, etc., for retaining it.]

PAINS IN THE STOMACH.

Since the collecting together the fore-mentioned accounts, I have met with a book written by Dr. Boerhaave, the present professor of physic at Leyden, in Holland, who affirms, that drinking water, made very warm, is a good remedy to pacify griping pains in the stomach; and that it is proper to bathe wounds in the face with it, when they come to be just healed, so that the place be kept continually wet, which I conceive is best done by applying often linen cloths wet, and binding them on till they begin to dry, for this will prevent scars. And he saith, that warm water is better to attenuate, or thin the blood, than cold water.

[Boerhaave, the greatest physician of his time, promulgated the theory that fever is caused by a *lentor* (something cold) in the blood. Hence his recommendation of warm water. It was through Boerhaave's doctrines that the heating treatment in fevers and inflammatory diseases became adopted, and to the destruction of thousands upon thousands within the last century. So much harm the mistake of an honest man may do.]

FEVERS.

There is also published lately a book of experiments made with water, by Dr. Hancock, a divine, called Febrifugum Mangum; wherein he saith, that drinking a pint or a quart of cold water in bed, will raise a copious sweat, and cure all burning fevers, which at once taking hath done the business. It will raise a sweat without much more covering than ordinary. And he further affirms, that the same taken at the beginning of the cold fit of an ague, and sweating upon it, at two or three times taking will cure that distemper. A large quantity of hot water, I know, hath been advised to take off the cold fit of agues, but the party was not ordered to sweat. Which discovery of the reverend doctor about fevers, is confirmed by the following accounts, which I received from a worthy gentleman, Mr. Ralph Thoresby, F. R. S.,* to whom they were transmitted by Mr. Lucas,

* Author of Ducatus Leediensis, or Topography of Leeds, which the learned Bishop of Lincoln, in his preface to the new edition of Camden's Britannia, styles an useful and accurate treatise.

a pious and learned gentleman of Leeds, in Yorkshire, who says:

"One Captain Rosier fell into a violent fever, which, as soon as he perceived, he said he must have some cold water. The gentlewoman at whose house he lodged, not thinking that proper, boiled the water (unknown to him) and put some spirits therein, and sent it up cold; but he smelt it before it came to his head, and refused to drink it, saying, he knew what he did, for he had several times tried it. Afterward some clear water being brought, he drank it, sweat profusely, and was well the next day.

"Another captain of a ship also took the same method, when he, or any of his men, fell into a fever; which had the desired success."

Mr. Lucas adds, in another letter to the same gentleman, "that his own wife fell very ill of a fever; she drank water, sweat very much, and thereby recovered."

All which instances corroborate the new way of curing fevers, so lately discovered in this city, by Dr. Hancock; who also saith, he has had long experience in curing common colds with cold water; and this is done by drinking a large draught of water at going to bed, another in the night, and another in the morning; which, he saith, will soon thicken, and sweeten, and digest that thin, sharp rheum, that provokes coughing to no purpose; for the rheum, when thin, is hard to be brought up, but when thickened, it will come up easily, and the cough will soon go off. Which agrees with what I before affirmed from my own long experience.

He also affirms from his own experience, that using sometimes to take a walk of eight or ten miles in a morning, he found that water gave twice as good breath for that purpose as wine or ale; and if it would do this for a man who had no asthma, he doubts not but it would do the same in one troubled with one. And he also affirms water to be the best remedy for a surfeit, to the truth of which I can testify by long experience.

RHEUMATISM.

He also affirms, that drinking cold water hath been found good in rheumatisms, and that to one so afflicted he had advised to drink it as he lay in his bed, and it took off the fit. But if hot water attenuates the blood most, as Boerhaave affirms, it is then best to drink of it warm daily to a good quantity; for, as Pitcairn observes, it is then the best dissolver of all kinds of salts in the body, which it will carry off in the urine, if drank plentifully; for by urine, salts are evacuated, as is evident by the taste.

[Warm water drank very freely is much better than none at all; but cold water is the best, provided no violence is done with it. Those who are feeble, and have long been accustomed to hot drinks, may commence with warm water, gradually coming to the cold, which will not require a long time. There are multitudes of dyspeptic, nervous persons, in our country, who would, in a few months, experience an amount of benefit far exceeding their most sanguine hopes, if they would but take resolutely to water, excluding every other drink.]

GOUT IN THE STOMACH.

And it is his opinion, from the long experience he hath had of the effect of water in keeping the stomach in order, and making it tight and strong to perform its operations, and digest all humors, that it will cure the gout in the stomach; and perhaps it may do it better than wine, which I have known to fail. And I do not wonder that the same liquor which is the principal cause of the gout in other parts, should not be a help in that part, but rather kill, as it often is found to do, though the strongest wine is drank.

In short, he affirms, and that with great reason, that sweating in fevers by drinking cold water, is more natural than to do it with hot sudorifics, which often do harm in the beginning of fevers, except good store of cooling, moistening liquors are drank with them, they being more apt to inflame that cool and quench heat in the body; and for that reason sweating hath not been often advised by physicians, because they were ignorant of this way of sweating to cure fevers, by drinking cold water.

Whicn cure, he said, did succeed in one who was his relation, at the fifth day after his falling sick; to whom he gave a dose of water after he was in bed, and he sweated profusely for twenty-four hours, and thereby was cured. Half a pint, he saith, is enough for a grown child: a pint to a man or woman, though if they drink a quart, it will be better. And in scarlet fevers, small-pox, or measles, though the water will not cause sweat, yet it will so quell and keep under the fever, that the eruptions will come out more kindly; which is a confirmation of what before was said about Dr. Betts' prescribing two quarts of water, when the small-pox did not come out kindly; the water affording matter to fill them up, according to what the author observes of a certain person, in the History of Cold Bathing (p. 347), that he could give an hundred instances where people of all ages have been lost by being denied drink in the small-pox; for it hinders the filling of the pustules.

PLAGUE.

And Dr. Hancock sets down an account of the author of the Free Thinker, concerning a woman, who, in the last great plague, fell ill of that distemper, who got her husband to fetch her a pitcher of water from Lamb's conduit: she drank plentifully of it, but did not avoid the cold, and so did not sweat; however, she was cured. And he gives us another relation of an Englishman, formerly resident at Morocco, that fell ill of the plague at that place, and getting water to drink, fell into a violent sweat, and recovered: from whence he concludes, that water is good in the plague; agreeable to what is related in Sir John Floyer's Book of Cold Baths, wherein it is said, that but two died of the plague who lived over the water upon London Bridge (p. 223), the coolness of the air being supposed to contribute to their health, who inhabited on the water in that manner, their blood being cooler than others: it is said, also, that watermen escaped better than others.

I will here add to what the doctor hath said before concerning the cure of fevers, that if the fever be accompanied in the beginning with any great illness at the stomach, nauseating or vomiting, it will be the surest and safest practice to clear the stomach first, by vomiting with warm water, as before hath been directed; for I cannot believe it possible for the stomach to be cleared from foul humors by sweating: it may do, if no great sense of disorder is perceived there, but it will certainly be safest to cleanse the stomach first, which is the place where all diseases are originally begun; for then sweating with cold water afterward may turn to good account. Indeed I have not made any trial of it since the doctor's book was published, but I have a very good opinion of his account therein given concerning the benefit of water, having had so much experience thereof in my own practice for above forty years; for so long it is since I first began to collect those accounts, and make those experiments, which are herein made public for the benefit of all.

And thus, for the common good of mankind, of all ranks and degrees, I have gathered together all the accounts I have observed in physic books relating to the use of common water in preventing and curing diseases; to which I have added some experiments of my own, which by numerous trials I can warrant as sure and certain, especially that of curing any sickness in the stomach upon the spot, by vomiting with warm water: which is an experiment, that, if put into common practice, would prevent many thousand fits of sickness in a year among mankind, and also a great number of untimely deaths; for it takes away the cause of all stomach sickness, which is the root or first beginning of most of the evils that afflict the body.

SOME RULES FOR PRESERVING HEALTH BY DIET, COLLECTED FROM AUTHORS OF PHYSIC.

In a little treatise, entitled, Kitchen Physic, written by Dr. Cook, the author declares, he can hardly be told of any disease which he cannot relieve or cure by a proper diet (p. 39). And in the same book we find his opinion to be this: that all tender, sickly people, and all aged and decrepit persons, ought to eat often, and but a little at a time, because weak and wasted bodies are to be restored by little and little; and by moist and liquid food also, rather than by solid, because moist and liquid diet does nourish soonest, and digest easiest.

Those, he saith, that eat much, and get little strength by eating, show that they have used themselves to too full a diet; and the more you cram such bodies, the less they thrive by it, but rather grow worse and worse: because, by much feeding, you do but add to the bad humors wherewith the body is already filled, which should rather be wasted by purging, and using a spare diet.

And a spare diet he describes to be this: that we never eat at once till the appetite is fully satisfied, and never to eat till we have an appetite; and men never have a true appetite till they can eat any ordinary food: and he adviseth to keep constantly to a plain diet; for those, he says, enjoy most health, and live longest, that avoid curiosity and variety of meats and drinks, which only serve to entice to gluttony, and so work our ruin.

Another faith, that the less food the sick person eats, the sooner he will recover; for it is a true saying, the more you fill foul bodies, the more you hurt them. The stomach being the place where diseases begin, when that part therefore is weak, and out of order, and cannot make a good digestion when much is eaten, raw or crude humors then must needs be bred, and bad humors cannot produce good blood.

All men do find by experience, that in the morning before they have eaten, they are light and pleasantly easy in their bodies, but after they have indulged their appetites with plenty of food, they find themselves heavy and dull, and often sleepy: which sufficiently shows that those full meals are prejudicial to the welfare of the body; for a moderate meal would have continued the ease and lightsomeness they before found in themselves, and would have refreshed any faintness that emptiness might occasion. And he certainly, who useth the most simple meats and drinks, avoideth the snare of provoking his appetite beyond the necessities of nature; whereas variety enticeth to a fresh desire of every dainty, till at last the stomach is gorged, and made uncapable of performing a good digestion; and this produceth those crudities, which are the cause of all diseases, and of so many sudden deaths.

It is generally observed, that the most unhealthy are found among those who feed high upon the most delicious dainties, and drink nothing but the strongest and most spirituous liquors; whereas, others who want this delicate fare, are seldom sick, except they have such unsatiable appetites as to eat too much, which a man may do of the plainest diet, whose belly is his god, as an apostle expresses it. But though men may glut themselves with coarse food, yet coarse food and long life are very consistent, as appears by John Bill, mentioned in the History of Cold Baths (p. 408), whose food was bread, cheese, and butter; and drink, whey, buttermilk or water; and yet he lived one hundred and thirty-three years, was a strong, straight, upright man. And the food of John Bailes, whose age amounted to one hundred and twenty-eight, was for the most part brown bread and cheese, and his drink water, or small beer and milk (p. 416). He had buried the whole town of Northampton twenty times over, except three or four, and said strong drink killed them all.

Dr. Pratt adviseth to sup sparingly; for to sup sparingly, he saith, is most healthful, because of the experience of an infinite number of persons who have received the greatest benefit from light suppers. For the stomach being not over-burdened, the sleep is more pleasant; and from sparing suppers the breeding of those humors are prevented, which cause defluxions, rheumatisms, gouts, dropsies, giddiness, and corruption in the mouth from the scurvy; and from light suppers a freedom from sickness and retching in the morning is obtained, and concoction is made perfect, which prevents obstructions.

Another saith, it is well-known that many indispositions are cured by fasting, or a very spare diet; for what is taken into the stomach being no more than can be well digested, the chylous juice, so rightly prepared, is conveyed into the lacteal vessels, and from thence into the blood: so that nature being duly supplied with well-concocted nourishment, the corrupted blood will free itself from that corruption in time, by throwing it out, through the pores of the skin, in perspiration, and supply itself with the purer juices; and in this way, consumptions and scurvies, and other chronical distempers, will be overcome; which way of curing diseases by fasting, swine do naturally betake themselves to, who, when sick, will eat nothing till they recover, as they always do after they injure themselves by over-eating; in which they are imitated by all who delight in gormandizing or gluttony, though not in using the same means of recovery.

That men in health may prevent diseases, it was advised that one meal should not be eaten till the other, which was eaten before, was passed off clean out of the stomach, which never is done till the appetite of hunger is found to call for another supply: by means of which constant observation, the food will be converted into good chyle, and from good chyle, which is a milky substance, good blood will be bred, and from good blood generous spirits will be produced, out of which a healthy constitution will ensue; but, on the contrary, too great a quantity of food being taken for pleasure only, which the stomach cannot well digest, the chyle will be raw and corrupt, which will foul the blood, and render the body disorderly and unhealthful.

Others say that abstinence and sobriety free from most diseases, especially catarrhs, coughs, wheezings, giddiness, pain in the head and stomach, sudden death, lethargies, gout, and sciatica, an ill digestion being the cause of all these; it also prevents pain in the spleen, stone, and gravel, and a dry itch; it makes the body vigorous and nimble, maintains the five senses in a good state, preserveth the memory, quickens the wit, and quencheth all undue lust in mankind; and, in short, all misers who eat and drink but little, live long.

Two meals a day is said to be sufficient for all persons after fifty years of age, and all weak people; and the omitting of suppers does always conduce much to health of the weak and aged, since if no supper be eaten, the stomach will soon free itself from all tough, slimy humors wherewith it is slabbered over on the inside, and thereby the appetite will be renewed, and digestion made more strong and vigorous. Moreover, all that are troubled with sweating in the night, any ill taste in their mouths, belching and troublesome dreams, must avoid suppers; for in sleep the fibres of the stomach relax, and are not able to contract themselves so strongly as when awake, to embrace the food, and by trituration reduce it into a pap fit to pass out into the other bowels, called the guts, out of which the nourishment is sent to other parts.

[Three meals a day, in proper quantity, are doubtless better than two. If those persons who eat but twice per day, would divide the same amount of food into three parts, taking the meals as nearly as might be at six, twelve, and six of the day, they will find it a better mode. But it must be acknowledged there is here a greater liability to take too much food.

Some persons have adopted the plan of eating but once in twenty-four hours, and are said to enjoy good health from such a practice. But we cannot regard this as a good one, for the most healthy desire food as often as three times a day. Three times a day, we have come to the conclusion from study and experiment, is the best general rule.]

It was said by Dr. Curtis, that though those who use a spare diet cannot well bear long labor, yet such people, when their exercise is suitable to their strength, do live longer than those of a robust constitution, that think large feeding adds strength; especially such as being strong, use no exercise proportionable to it, to consume the superfluities which a full feeding doth occasion; so that the only way for those to live long who have much wealth, and need not labor for a livelihood, is to live temperately; and this temperance doth consist in not letting the common custom of meals invite you to eat, except your appetite concur with those times. We must not indulge the cravings of a depraved appetite, as those do who eat to please their fancy, and not the necessities of nature; and when we do eat, we must not think that the more plentifully we eat, we shall be more strengthened, for it will not prove so; a little well digested will make the body stronger, than the being glutted with superfluity, most of which will be turned into a corrupt juice, and must be cast out by physic, or else sickness will ensue, and the easiest physic is that which the Germans call the hunger-cure, if continued a due time.

It is the opinion of learned men, that the early distemper of the bodies of children, called the rickets, proceeds from the fault of their mothers, in making them gluttons from their cradles, gorging them with food till they loath it, out of a mistaken opinion that this is the way to make them thrive and grow strong; which excess is not only the cause of this disease, but of the immature death of many; and in others it lays the foundation of many distempers, which afflict those afterward who live to the years of maturity; and as they gorge them with food, so they vainly think to cherish them with strong drink, than which nothing can be more pernicious to the health of children, whose diet should be little and often, and their drink cooling. As it also should be when men arrive at the time of becoming children again in old age; that is, in an helpless state, which should be prevented as much as can be, by a cooling, moistening diet, in opposition to the hot, and dry, and withered state of age; for it is heat and dryness that are the cause of most old men's miseries, especially the wasting of the substance that fills the parts with moisture, and keeps the body plump and smooth; they who style wine the old man's milk, being greatly mistaken, for milk cools, and wine heats.

It was the opinion of Dr. Pitt, who was formerly physician to St. Bartholomew's Hospital, that fasting, rest, and drinking water, would cure most diseases; and there seemeth to be a great deal of reason in what he asserted. For fasting will give time to the stomach to unload itself of the cause of distempers, the cause of all diseases being begun in that bowel only; to which cleansing, the drinking of water plentifully will much contribute, which also will keep the action of the stomach upon the hinges, by filling of it when empty, at which time there will be need of rest, for thereby the body will be less fit for business: though the mere drinking of water, which affords nourishment sufficient for the growth and support of all vegetables, will, in some measure, supply the want of food, as hath been shown in the example of two, who were supported a long time by nothing else. In short, the best way for a sick man to recover, is to eat little or no food till he finds an appetite, according to that saying,

> "Spare diet will the most diseases cure,
> If a due time you can the same endure."

And fasting from food may be continued long enough to be a remedy for many diseases, with the assistance of common water: by drinking of which warm, in a due quantity, without a total fasting, two persons, I am informed, were recovered out of consumptions, with which they were extremely weakened, and that in about six weeks' time; as was another by drinking milk and whey, equal parts, made blood-hot, without using any other diet, which is thought to be far more effectual than asses' milk, whose virtue consists in being thinner than other milk.

But besides a spare diet, cool, dry air is also very helpful to preserve men in health, who are not sick, for it mixes with the blood, and without it the motion of the blood and spirits can never be preserved, as appears by diving vessels, in which men cannot live when the air therein is made hot by their own body and breath: and is proved, also, by an experiment of Dr. Croone's, who stifled a chicken, till it seemed quite dead; and yet by blowing cool air into the lungs, with a small pair of bellows, it revived. Hence it appears, that the common custom of managing sick people is very pernicious, and so far from helping them to recover, that it is sufficient to make a healthy person sick; for were a person, who was not sick, confined for three or four weeks in a room, made hot like a stove, and kept in his bed, with the curtains drawn, and all the windows close shut, and the room made unpleasant with the nauseous fumes of physic, and a close stool, which will almost make a fresh man sick when he just enters into it; we can never think that this is the way to recover one that really is sick, and wants the fresh air and reviving scents to cherish his blood; a fresh, open, sweet air being one principal means to strengthen the body, make a good appetite and digestion, and render the spirits brisk and lively: which advantage should be allowed to all but child-bed women, and those who are afflicted with the small-pox; for the fresh air can be prejudicial to no other, whose bodies are clothed warm, either in bed, or sitting in a chair in their chamber.

Some years since a neighbor became very feverish, and his wife persuaded him to go to bed; and hearing of it soon after, I gave him a visit, where I found the windows close shut, the curtains of the bed drawn, and the room very hot, for it was in July: he was burning hot, and complained for want of breath. I drew open the curtains, covered him warm, and then opened the windows, and the wind blew into the room; upon which he soon told me, his shortness of breath had left him. I persuaded him to drink some water, which he found did much refresh him; and after I had taken my leave of him, he called for more water: and while he had the cup in his hand, an apothecary came in, whom his wife had sent for, who, finding him about to drink the water, told him, if he did it he was a dead man; but instead of forbearing, he drank it up in his presence: upon which the other took his leave, and told him, he would say no more to him. However, before night, the person got up, went abroad, and was cured of his fever; which is one instance, among many others that might be given, of the benefit of fresh air to a person who is kept warm in his bed; for thereby his body was cooled inwardly, and his breathing made more free, by the air which was drawn into his lungs to refresh and comfort the blood as it passed through them.

I shall only add, that by keeping the blood cool as well as clean, is to be understood, not only moderation in diet, but to feed most on cooling food made of wheat, barley, oatmeal, rice, and ripe apples, as also on milk; which, joined with oatmeal, is the chief food of those lusty and strong men, the Highlanders of Scotland, who abound in children, as Dr. Cheyne tells us, in his Treatise of the Gout (p. 108, edit. iv.), which demonstrates milk and oatmeal to be a most strengthening food, and such as keeps the blood in due order; so that therewith men may subsist, though they abstain from beef, pork, and venison, and all other meats hard to digest, and drink water as the Highlanders do: of the efficacy of which cooling milk diet, the said Dr. Cheyne gives a notable instance in a doctor that lived at Croyden (p. 103), who had long been afflicted with the falling-evil; for, by slow observation, he found the lighter his meals were, the lighter were his fits. At last he also cast off all liquids but water, and found his fits weaker, and the intervals longer; and finding his disease mend, as its fuel was withdrawn, he took to vegetable food and water only, which put an entire period to his fits without any relapse: but finding that food windy to him, he took to milk, of which he eat a pint for breakfast, a quart at dinner, and a pint for supper, without fish, flesh, bread, or any strong or spirituous liquor, or any drink but water, with which he lived afterward for fourteen years, without the least interruption in his health, strength, or vigor, but died afterward of a pleurisy. Which is a confirmation of what Dr. Cook did affirm, of the possibility of curing diseases by diet only that is temperate and cooling.

In short, temperance or a spare diet, void of dainties, never was injurious to the strongest constitution, and without it, such as are weak and sickly cannot long subsist; for the more such persons eat and drink, the more weak and disordered they will still find themselves to be: so that if the strong despise temperance, yet the comfort of weak, sickly, and pining people, does depend entirely upon their constantly observing it; which, when they are accustomed to it, will be easy to do: so that they will deny all intemperate desires with as great pleasure, as they before did delight in what is falsely styled good eating and drinking; for nothing of that is good which is injurious to health; it is custom only that makes men hanker after gluttony and drunkenness, and a contrary custom will make men abhor it as much. And therefore it is a wonder the rich do not strive to attain to it, for

> "A fatal error 'tis, in men of wealth,
> To feed so high as will destroy their health."

Temperance being that which will enable them to live most at ease, and enjoy their wealth the longest; this, and water-drinking, being the surest way to bring men to old age, though it hath not power to make the aged young.

APPENDIX

INNUTRITIOUS MATTER IN FOOD NECESSARY TO HEALTH.

It is a well ascertained law of the animal economy, that food, to be healthy, must contain a considerable portion of matter that is wholly indigestible and innutritious. Thus, Magendie, the physiologist, found that dogs, fed upon sugar, gum arabic, butter, olive oil, and some other articles of rich or concentrated nature, each given to the animals separately with pure water, they very soon lost their appetites, began to droop, became emaciated, were attacked with ulcers, and died, invariably, within the space of four or five weeks. Fed upon superfine flour-bread and water, they lived uniformly about seven weeks, varying only a day or two. When fed upon coarse or military bread, such as contained either the whole or a considerable portion of the bran, the dogs thrived perfectly well, and were found in no respect to suffer. The same truth has often been illustrated upon ship-board at sea. In many cases, where the hay and straw were swept overboard, it has been found that the animals, in a few days, famished, unless some innutritious substance, as the shavings of wood, was mixed with the grain given them. The animals have been observed to gnaw at the spars and timbers, or whatever wood they could lay hold of; and thus the idea was suggested, that the grain alone was of too rich a nature for their sustenance.

The same principle holds good in reference to the health of the human body, and as a general fact, food, in civilized life, is of too concentrated a quality. This is particularly true in those parts of the world where an abundance can be had; in other words, in the more civilized and enlightened parts of the world. A host of diseases, both acute and chronic, are either caused or greatly aggravated by concentration in food. Indigestion, with its immense train of evils, constipation, loss of flesh, corpulency, nervous and general debility, torpor, and sluggishness of the general system, are the principal roots of all disease in the human family, and these are among the difficulties caused by too great richness in food. Children are often injured in this way. Mothers, in their kindness, think nothing too good for their little ones. In many parts of our country, the infant at the breast is taught to suck at its piece of pork, or other fat meat. Sugar, sugar candy, sweetened milk, superfine bread, and rich pastries, are all given for the same reason, by mothers and nurses in their mistaken kindness. Children reared in this way can never be healthy for any considerable length of time, are generally very puny and weak, and often die within two or three years of birth. Scrofulous and other ulcers are frequently thus caused, and so also those derangements of the stomach and bowels, which so often, in spite of the best remedial means, sweep these little sufferers from their earthly existence, and this at the very time when their growing mind begins to gladden the parent's heart. There is great and prevailing error upon this subject, and happy are those parents who take it upon themselves to gain wisdom in this most important matter of food.

Sedentary and studious persons, and especially young ladies at seminaries and boarding-schools, suffer much from the effects of superfine bread, and other forms of concentrated food. Constipation, which is always attended with unpleasant results, is very common among this class of persons, one of the greatest causes of that state of health being too great richness in food.

The effects of superfine flour were strikingly illustrated in the case of a crew of seamen belonging to Providence, R. I. The narrative we quote from Graham's Science of Human Life, and is as follows:

"Captain Benjamin Dexter, of the ship Isis, belonging to Providence, R. I., arrived from China, in December, 1804. He had been about one hundred and ninety days on the passage. The sea-bread, which constituted the principal article of food for his hands, was made of the best of superfine flour. He had not been long at sea, before the men began to complain of languor, loss of appetite, and debility. These difficulties continued to increase during the whole voyage, and several of the men died on the passage, of debility and inanition. The ship was obliged to come to anchor about thirty miles below Providence; and such was the debility of the hands on board, that they were not able to get the ship under way again; and the owners were under the necessity of sending men down from the city of Providence to work her up. When she arrived, the owners asked Capt. Dexter what was the cause of the sickness of his men, to which he answered, 'The bread is too good.'"

Cases of a similar kind have elsewhere been known to occur. Sailors, the world over, are generally furnished with brown sea-bread, much to the advantage of this useful class of men, did they but know it; and their health is proverbially good while they are away from the temptations upon land. These hardy, weather-beaten men are subjected to many healthful influences other than the use of coarse bread, but, on the whole, their dietetic and other hygienic habits need greatly to be improved ; still, compared with the mass of mankind, they are remarkably healthy.

Every one who is aware of the importance of a certain degree of innutritiousness in food, must lament many of the so-called improvements of modern times. Who can think of the good dishes our New England mothers used to prepare, homely and plain, as the fastidious would now consider them to be, and not desire earnestly that such days of simplicity might again return to us? As things are, if a person travels from home, or visits among friends, almost every dish that is set before him is of a form so concentrated as to be positively injurious. At the best hotels and boarding-houses, upon the floating palaces that glide upon our waters, and in our splendid ships that traverse the seas, the evil we speak of is generally prevalent.

POTATOES A PREVENTIVE AND CURE FOR SCURVY.

Much has been said of late, in France and England, of the value of this vegetable in the prevention and cure of scorbutic disease, administered several times a day in its *raw state*, but scraped sufficiently fine to make it digestible. It seems to have been amply tested among the seamen of the French navy. In the United States army, this is no new remedy in scorbutus. Thus, in the first quarter of 1821, there were sixteen cases reported at Fort Crawford, Prairie du Chien, of which two terminated fatally. The medical officer, in his report, according to the "statistics of the United States Army," speaking of the employment of "*raw potatoes and vinegar*," says: "I selected four or five of the worst cases, which had received no alleviation from the use of the nitre and vinegar, and directed each one to eat, per day, a common soup-plate full of the potato, sliced down in a sufficient quantity of vinegar. It had an immediate effect on the stomach, which recovered its natural vigor; the bowels became regular, the pains abated, the stricture of the tendons was overcome, the ulcers put on a healthy aspect, and in a few days the patient found himself in a happy state of convalescence."—*The New York Journal of Medicine for July, edited by S. Forry, M. D.*

POTATOES AS A DIET—EXPERIMENTS AT THE GLASGOW BRIDEWELL, IN 1840.

Breakfast.—Eight ounces of oatmeal made into porridge, with a pint of buttermilk.

Dinner.—Three pounds of boiled potatoes with salt.

Supper.—Five ounces of oatmeal made into porridge, with half a pint of buttermilk.

Ten prisoners, five men and five boys, were placed upon this diet, having been previously examined relative to their health, and weighed. They were employed in light work, and under sentence of confinement for two months. At the beginning of the experiment, eight were in good health, and two in indifferent health; at the end, all were in good health, and they had, on an average, gained more than four pounds each in weight, only one prisoner, a man, having lost in weight. The greatest gain was nine pounds four ounces, and was made by one of the men; the prisoner who was reduced in weight had lost five pounds two ounces. *Cost*, including cooking, 2¾d. It was found by experiment, that baked potatoes were far less nourishing than boiled, the prisoners losing, on an average, 1½ pounds weight, instead of gaining, though in all other respects the diet was the same as in the former experiment. The addition of a quarter of a pound of meat to the diet did not add to their weight; on the contrary, the prisoners lost, on an average, 1¼ pounds. The results were not more satisfactory when the quantity of meat was increased to half a pound at dinner. In an experiment upon the same number of persons, the diet consisted as follows:

Breakfast.—Two pounds of potatoes boiled.

Dinner.—Three pounds of potatoes boiled.

Supper.—One pound of potatoes boiled.

At the beginning of the experiment, eight were in good health, and two in indifferent health; at the end, the eight continued in good health, and the two who had been in indifferent health had improved. There was, on an average, a gain in weight of nearly 3½ pounds per prisoner, the greatest gain being 8¼ pounds. Only two lost in weight, and the quantity in each case was trifling. The prisoners all expressed themselves satisfied with this diet, and regretted the change back again to the ordinary diet. On the whole, these experiments prove that prisoners may be kept in good condition at a very moderate expense, the cost not exceeding 6d. per day, when fed as above. Indeed, we know, from an experiment conducted on a still larger scale in Ireland, that potatoes and milk, with a little oatmeal, are sufficient for healthy nutrition.—*Fifth Report of the Inspectors of Prisons in Scotland, by Frederick Hill,* 1840.

INDEX.

ALPHABETICAL LIST OF BOOKS

PUBLISHED BY

FOWLERS AND WELLS,

NO. 131 NASSAU ST., NEW YORK.

American Phrenological Journal and Miscellany Circulation, 20,000 copies. A year, - $1 00

A Home for All; or, a New, Cheap, Convenient, and Superior Mode of Building, - - - - 50

Amativeness; or, Evils and Remedies of Excessive and Perverted Sexuality, with Advice, - - 12½

A Manual for Magnetizing with the Magnetic Machine, for the Treatment of Disease, - - - 50

Botany for all Classes; Containing a Floral Dictionary, with more than One Hundred Illustrations, 50

Combe's Lectures on Phrenology. By George Combe. A complete course. With Illustrations, 1 00

Constitution of Man, considered in Re-lation to External Objects. Revised and enlarged edition, - 50

Combe's Physiology, applied to the Im-provement of Mental and Physical Education, - - - - 50

Combe on Infancy; or, the Physiologi-cal and Moral Management of Children. Illustrated, - - 50

Consumption, its Prevention and Cure, by the Water Treatment. By Joel Shew, M.D., - - - 50

Chronic Diseases, especially the Nerv-ous Diseases of Women. Dy D. Rosch, - - - 25

Curiosities of Common Water. With Additions by Joel Shew, M.D. From the 5th London edition, 25

Cholera; its Causes, Prevention, and Cure; and all other Bowel Complaints, treated by Water, - 25

Chemistry, Applied to Physiology, Ag-riculture, and Commerce. By Professor Liebig, - - - 20

Chart, for Recording various Developments. Designed for Phrenologists, - - - - - - 6¼

Defence of Phrenology. By Dr. Andrew Boardman. A good work for skeptics and unbelievers, - 50

Education Complete. Embracing Physiology, Animal and Mental, Self-Culture, and Memory, - - 2 00

Education, founded on the Nature of Man. By Dr. Spurzheim. A scientific work, - - - 50

Familiar Lessons on Phrenology. Designed for the use of Children and Youth, - - 50

Food and Diet: Containing an Analysis of every kind of Food and Drink. By Professor Pereira, 50

Fascination, or the Philosophy of Charming. (Magnetism.) Illustrating the Principles of Life, 40

Familiar Lessons on Astronomy: Designed for Children and Youth in Schools and Families, - - 40

Familiar Lessons on Physiology. Designed for the use of Children and Youth, . - - - 25

Hereditary Descent: its Laws and Facts applied to Human Improvement. New edition, - 50

Human Rights, and their Political Guaranties By Judge Hurlbut. With Notes by George Combe 50

Hydropathy for the People, with Observations on Drugs, Diet, Water, Air, Exercise, etc., - 50

Love and Parentage: applied to the Improvement of Offspring, - - - - - - 25

Lectures on the Philosophy of Mesmerism and Clairvoyance, with Instruction in its Process, - 25

Moral and Intellectual Science. By Combe, Stratton, Cox, Gregory, and others. Illustrated, - 2 00

Maternity: or, the Bearing and Nursing of Children, including Female Education, - - 50

Memory and Intellectual Improvement: Applied to Self-Education and Juvenile Instruction, - - 50

Mesmerism in India. A Superior work, by the celebrated Dr. Esdaile, - - - - - 50

Marriage: its History and Philosophy, with an Exposition of the Functions of Happy Marriages, - 37½

Matrimony: or, Phrenology and Physi-ology applied to the Selection of Companions for Life, - - 25

Natural Laws of Man, Physiologically Considered. By Dr. Spurzheim. A good work, - - - 25

Phrenology Proved, Illustrated, and Ap-plied. Thirty-seventh edition, in muslin, - - - - - 1 00

Physiology, Animal and Mental: Ap-plied to Health of Body and Power of Mind, - - - 50

Power of Kindness; Inculcating the Christian Principles of Love over Physical Force, - - - 25

Popular Phrenology, exhibiting the Phrenological Developments of more than fifty persons, - - 25

Physiology of Digestion, considered with Relation to the Principles of Dietetics. Illustrated. - 25

Psychology, or the Science of the Soul. With Illustrations of the Brain and Nervous System, - - 25

Phrenological Guide: Designed for the Use of Students of their own Characters, - - - - - 12½

Phrenological Almanac: illustrated with numerous Engravings. A handsome Annual, - - - 6¼

Religion, Natural and Revealed: or the Natural Theology and Moral Bearings of Phrenology, - 50

Self-Culture and Perfection of Charac-ter, including the Management of Youth, - - - - - 50

Symbolical Head and Phrenological Chart, in Map Form, showing the Language of the Organs, - 25

Sober and Temperate Life: with Notes and Illustrations by John Burdell, - - - - 25

Self-Instructor in Phrenology and Physiology. Illustrated with One Hundred Engravings, - 25

Synopsis of Phrenology and Physiology; With Illustrations in Neurology - - - 12½

Science of Swimming: giving the History of Swimming, and Instruction to Learners, - - - 12½

The Parent's Guide, and Childbirth made Easy. By Mrs. Hester Pendleton, - - - - - - 50

Tobacco: its Effects on the Body and Mind. The best work on the subject, - - - - - - 25

Teeth: their Structure, Disease, and Management. By John Burdell, Dentist, - - - 12½

Temperance and Tight-Lacing; founded on the Laws of Life, - - - - - - - - 12½

Vegetable Diet, as Sanctioned by Medical Men, and Experience in All Ages, - - - 50

Water-Cure Journal and Herald of Reforms. Devoted to Hydropathy. A Health Journal. - - 1 00

Water-Cure Manual; a Popular Work on Hydropathy. By Joel Shew, M.D., - - - 50

Water-Cure in Every Known Disease. By J. H. Rausse. Translated by Dr. Meeker, - - - - 50

Water-Cure---Errors of Physicians and Others in the Application of. By J. H. Rausse, - - - 25

Water-Cure---Experience in. By Mrs. M. S. Gove Nichols. With Instructions in Water-Cure, - 25

Water-Cure for Women in Pregnancy and Childbirth. Illustrated with numerous cases, - - 25

Water-Cure Almanac, containing much important matter for the healthy and the unhealthy. Yearly. 6¼

Water and Vegetable Diet. By Wm. Lamb, M.D. From the London Edition, - - - - 50

Woman: her Education and Influence. With an Introduction by Mrs. Kirkland. Illustrated, - - 40

EITHER OF THESE WORKS may be ordered and received by return of the FIRST MAIL, at a trifling expense for postage. Please address, post-paid,

FOWLERS AND WELLS,
131 Nassau st., New York.

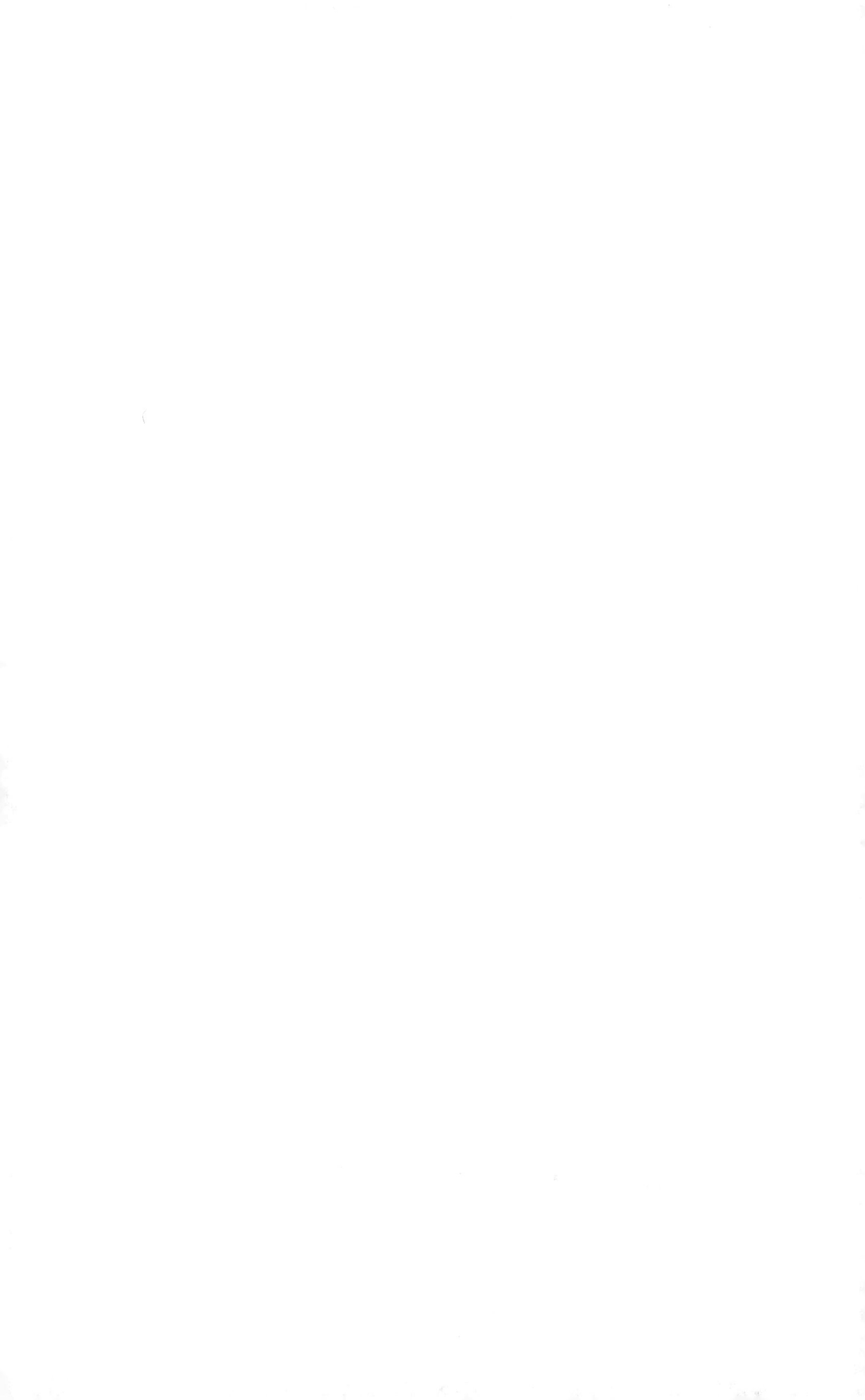

www.ingramcontent.com/pod-product-compliance
Lightning Source LLC
LaVergne TN
LVHW010208110826
845151LV00002B/640
* 9 7 8 1 4 2 5 5 3 5 7 3 5 *